THE 12-WEEK
TRIATHLETE

THE 12-WEEK
TRIATHLETE

Train for a Triathlon in Just Three Months
SPRINT · OLYMPIC · HALF-IRONMAN · IRONMAN

TOM HOLLAND

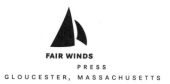

FAIR WINDS
PRESS
GLOUCESTER, MASSACHUSETTS

First published in the USA in 2005 by
Fair Winds Press
33 Commercial Street
Gloucester, MA 01930

2 3 4 5 6   09 08 07 06 05

ISBN 1-59233-126-2

Library of Congress Cataloging-in-Publication Data available

Cover design by Poul Hans Lange
Book design by *tabula rasa* graphic design
Photography by Allan Penn

Printed and bound in USA

This book is dedicated to my amazing wife, Philippa.

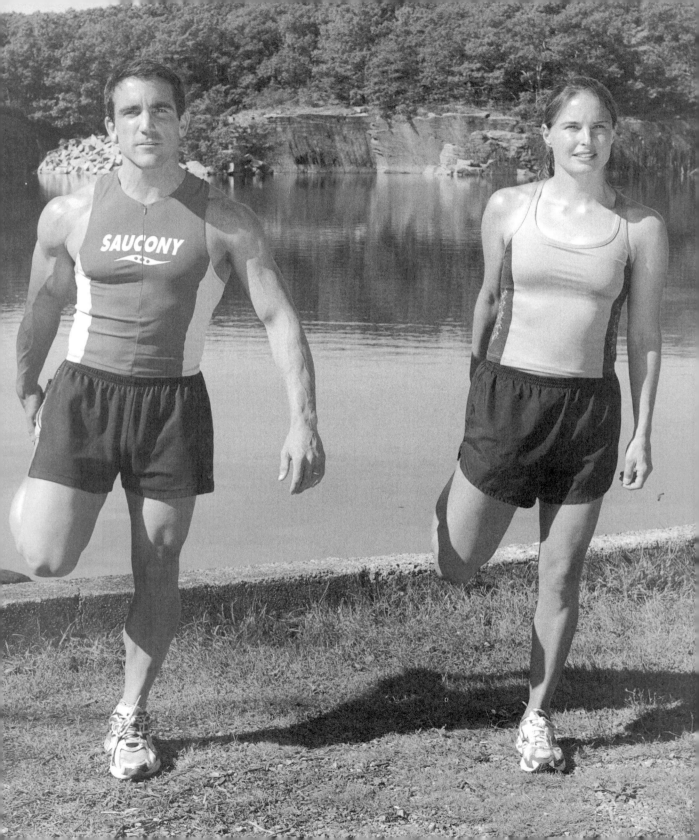

ACKNOWLEDGMENTS

Thank you to my father for taking me running when I was ten and for continuing to run with me ever since. And thank you to my mother for telling me I had skinny legs, which motivated me to begin lifting weights.

Special thanks to Troy Jacobson, from whom I learned a tremendous amount about the sport of triathlon, coaching, and making my passion my vocation; to bike guru Kevin Skeen for making my bike "scary fast" for my first Ironman; to Pat and his team at Northeast Bicycles for all their great bike support; and to Nicholas Broskovich for allowing me to chase him during his ridiculously long runs and bike workouts.

I am forever grateful to Dr. David Kemler for opening up to me the world of sports psychology, and to Dr. Donald Carone, who taught me the power of believing in yourself.

Additional thanks to all my clients who trusted me to guide them to the finish line.

Finally, thank you to my wife, Philippa, for her unending support in all of my endeavors, regardless of how big or how far.

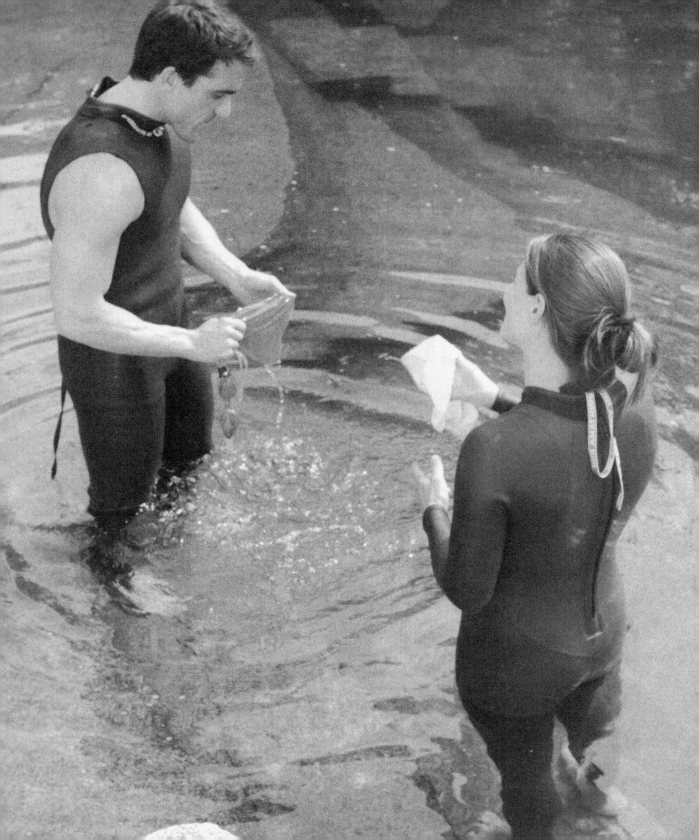

CONTENTS

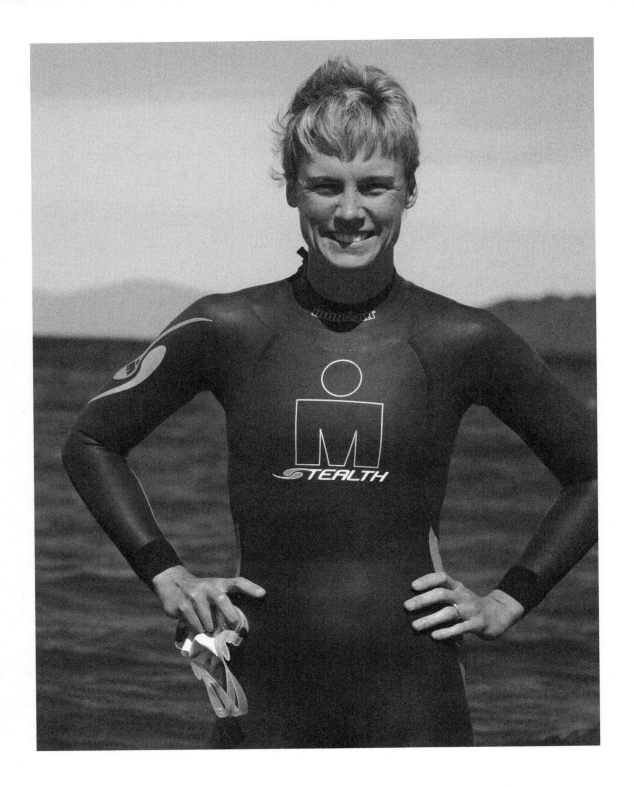

FOREWORD

Love it! *The 12-Week Triathlete,* by Tom Holland, is one of the best information and training resources I have come across for beginner to intermediate triathletes. The sport of triathlon can be intimidating, especially to the newcomer. There are many views on how to train using specific zones and what type of high-tech gear you absolutely need to get started. This alone can scare anyone from entering the sport and completing their first race. Tom eliminates all the fluff and unnecessary items in order to help athletes enjoy the sport and complete their goals. He explains everything—from proper core strength work and training schedules to what type of bike and wheel size you can use.

As a professional triathlete and coach, I adhere to the philosophies that Tom uses in his practice. The key to success with this sport is to remain healthy, enjoy what you are doing, and grow both as a person and as an athlete. By incorporating these themes into your training, not only will your fitness be elevated, but your overall value of life will be enhanced, and that is the richest reward of all.

Andrea Fisher
Professional Triathlete
Austin, Texas USA
www.andreafisher.com

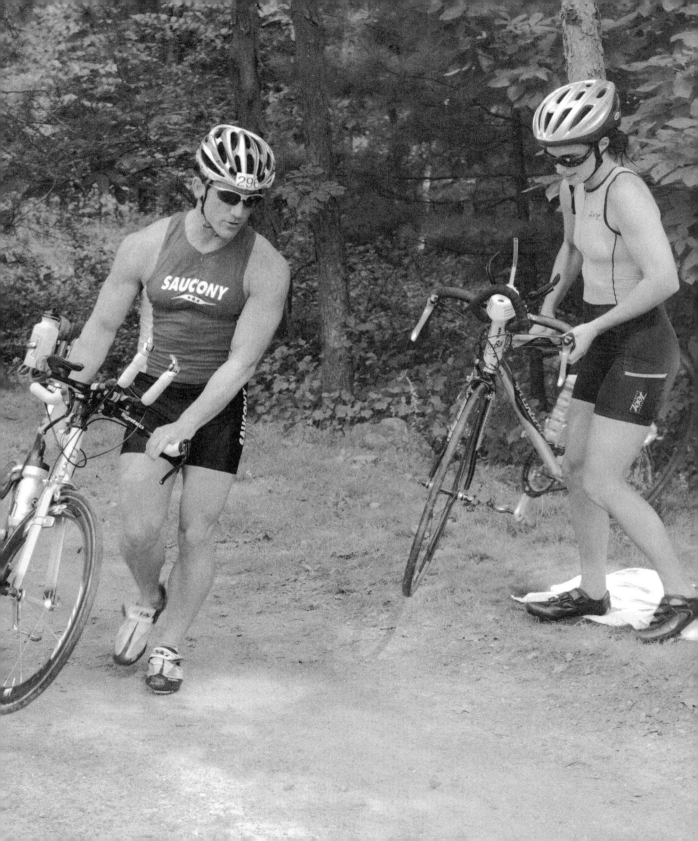

INTRODUCTION

Swim, bike, and run. Sounds like a perfect summer day's activities back when you were about eight years old. Well, some years ago, a group of Californians decided to combine these three great activities into one sport, and triathlon was born. Since then, the sport has exploded in popularity and it looks as if this trend will continue for many years to come. In this book I will do two simple things: first, I'll show you how to train for a triathlon, and second, I'll teach you what to do on race day. I will do this while adhering to three things that I consider to be paramount to lifelong success in triathlon, and to fitness, for that matter: staying injury-free, enjoying both training and competition, and improving yourself along the way. And no, you don't have to devote your life to training for your triathlon. I will outline twelve-week training programs that will fit into your life and get you to that start line healthy and ready to race.

Before I begin, I would like to share with you my first experience with the sport of triathlon. What I have discovered from talking to other triathletes over the years is that the story of my first race is far from unique.

MY FIRST TRI

My first triathlon was the Central Park Sprint Tri in New York City. At the time, I was a full-time personal trainer and group fitness instructor at several different gyms in Manhattan. While I had grown up running road races and had finished several marathons by that time, I truly had no idea what triathlons were all about. I had never even owned a real bike, unless you count the blue one I rode as a kid, complete with the banana seat. I had also never really swam except for yearly summer vacations at the beach, where I would practice my body-surfing technique rather than my freestyle stroke. But I love new challenges, and when I saw the flyer for this yearly event, I signed up. I rented a bike and a helmet, I purchased some cheap swim goggles, and I was ready.

Or so I thought.

After renting the bike I walked it home because, yes, I was too afraid to ride it through the streets of New York. It had all these gears and special cages for my feet (not even clip-ons!), two things I had absolutely no experience with. I pushed it down by the river where people walked and rollerbladed, and I felt safe attempting to learn how to ride this new-fangled machine. As I pedaled it up and down a few-hundred-yard straightaway and became more comfortable with it, I was hooked instantly. I can still remember how incredible it felt to ride. I rode it for thirty minutes or so and felt like a pro as I walked it back to my apartment. That was the extent of my bike training.

Race day. The swim was to be held in Lasker Pool in Central Park, and thus this was where the race check-in was and the transition area as well. As I approached the pool, it became increasingly evident that I didn't really look like the other competitors. Their bikes were different, with strange handlebars and funny-looking pedals; they were dressed much differently than I was, in tight-fitting clothes; and they were busy setting up their areas around bike racks. I watched the others around me and did what they did as far as assembling my preassigned area, but somehow it just didn't look like everyone else's. I seemed to be missing certain things that most people had, and had other things that no one else was using.

SWIM OR RUN?

And so I stood next to the pool in anticipation of the swim and my first triathlon start. Just a quarter of a mile swim, a handful of laps, no problem, I had thought. In the application, it had asked how fast you thought you would complete the swim portion, which I would later learn was to put you in the appropriate group. Having absolutely no idea because I didn't swim laps in a pool, I looked online at the results from the previous year's race and chose a time a little better than the average. Fast forward to my swim. As the gun went off, I swam

as hard as I could and made it (almost) halfway across the pool before I felt as if I were going to die. My lungs were screaming, I couldn't breathe, I was completely exhausted, and there was no way I could make it to the other side, much less swim the rest of the way. I stood up in the four feet of water and looked around, trying desperately to catch my breath. I noticed the person in the lane to my left had stopped as well to adjust his goggles, so I pretended to do the same. I walked a few steps and observed this person dive back in, swim a few lengths, and then stand again, cursing and running as he readjusted his obviously leaky goggles. I now had my strategy on how I would complete the swim without needing mouth-to-mouth resuscitation. The pool was four feet deep all the way across, and I would swim a stroke or two, stand and curse as I fixed my goggles while running several yards, then repeat until I had completed my swim leg. My ego was a little bruised, but I was alive and ready to take on part two, the bike. And, as I would slowly discover, the worst was over.

"HAMMERING" THE BIKE? NOT QUITE...

I managed to get through the transition area and onto my bike without much difficulty. I did notice that most people were using special shoes that attached onto pedals that looked nothing like mine. I was using the sneakers I planned on running in with cages on my pedals. Those cages were difficult enough for me to deal with; I couldn't imagine what it must be like to ride with that other type of shoe.

The twelve-mile bike entailed two loops of Central Park. As I began to pedal my tank of a rental bike along, it soon became evident that

I wasn't very fast. It seemed as if I was practically standing still as biker after biker whizzed by me. I struggled to get up the one hill in Harlem and felt spent at the top. I'll never forget the guy walking his dog along the side of the road who, as he watched me lumber by, yelled out, "Next time, get the right gear!" To this day I'm still not sure what he was specifically referring to, but now I was not only completely fatigued after just a few miles, but thanks to his comments, I was also self-conscious. Then a woman many years my senior hammered past me on a mountain bike, which didn't help matters one bit.

After what seemed like an eternity, I finally completed my two loops and made my way back to the transition area, which was now full of bikes, yet again reinforcing how darn slow I was moving. I was eternally grateful to get off that bike and was actually looking forward to the final leg, the run.

"WADDLING" THROUGH THE RUN

Now, as I stated earlier, I had run since I was about ten years old, hundreds of races, including several marathons. I considered myself to be a runner. But as I dismounted the bike and set off in the direction of the run course, something felt seriously wrong. My legs felt like lead, and I was running as if I had had a major accident in my pants. I had never run after having biked before, and this was now no secret to the group of spectators who watched as I waddled out onto the run course to begin the final five-kilometer run.

After a few minutes, my legs began to loosen up and my form began to slowly resemble that of normal running. I was still going slowly, mind you; I couldn't have run any faster if I had wanted desperately to, but I was running. And that's when I really began to reflect on what I had just accomplished and what I was about to complete, and I really began to enjoy myself. As I rounded the turn to the finish and saw my girlfriend cheering me on, a huge smile spread across my face and I knew that I had found my new sport.

Since then, I have competed in numerous sprint, Olympic, and Half-Ironman distance triathlons. I have completed ten Ironman distance triathlons, including ones in Malaysia, New Zealand, Australia, Germany and South Korea. I am injury-free, I love my training and racing, and I improve something each and every day I train. As a sports-performance coach, I have trained hundreds of people to successfully complete triathlons of all distances, using the same philosophy and techniques that are outlined in this book.

If you are considering doing your first triathlon, congratulations. What I tell clients who are in this "contemplative" stage is that they need to do two things: first, sign up for the race, then immediately tell ten friends that you are planning on doing it. This invests you in the process, both financially and emotionally. Spend the money on the race fee and tell those friends whom you would rather die than hear say, "I knew you weren't going to do it" if you decided to pull out of the race.

Maybe you have already participated in triathlons without much guidance, and now you want more specific direction. Maybe you became injured while training, perhaps you want to jump to a longer distance, or maybe you want to better your performances at triathlons of the same distance. This book will help you do all of those things, and if you follow it completely and consistently, it will absolutely get you into the best shape of your life.

I will outline training plans for the four major distances of triathlon: the sprint, Olympic, Half-Ironman, and Ironman distance races. I will provide you with two different types of training plans for each distance triathlon—"Finish" and "Performance" plans.

Finish: This category is for those who merely wish to finish their respective race. This would include first-time triathletes as well as those who are jumping up to compete in a longer-distance triathlon. My goal with each

of these plans is to get you to the start line healthy, have you fit enough that you enjoy the race, and do this without having the training dominate your life.

Performance: These four plans are designed for those who find that simply finishing your triathlon is not enough. You have most likely either competed in a few tris and wish to better your times, or you are a first-timer (newbie!) who has some idea of a time goal that you would like to attain. These plans have a higher volume (number and duration) of workouts than the Finish plans do, and incorporate speed into certain workouts.

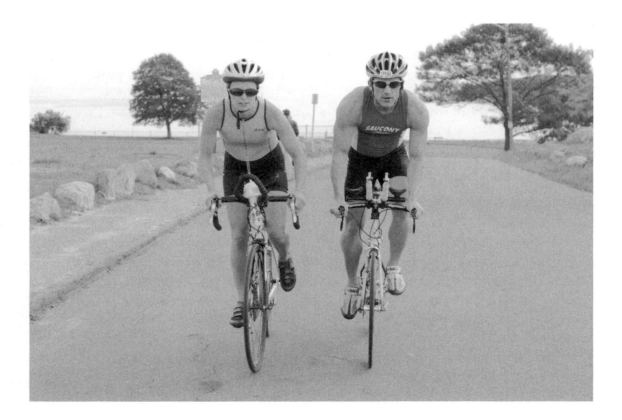

★ IMPORTANT NOTES

• While I could have written a book chock full of technical jargon and complex training plans that involve two- or three-a-day workouts along with numerous heart-rate zones, I have purposely chosen not to. It has been my personal experience that the vast majority of age-group athletes simply do not need this level of complexity when it comes to training and performing exceptionally within their abilities.

• Twelve weeks is indeed a relatively short amount of time to prepare for the longer-distance triathlons, including the Half-Ironman and Ironman distances. You can do it, but to do it effectively requires that you strictly adhere to all aspects of the plan—nutritional, strength training, flexibility, rest days, as well as the actual swim, bike, and run schedules. Those of you who will be following the Half-Ironman- and Ironman-distance programs should have a significant fitness base before attempting these races within this time frame.

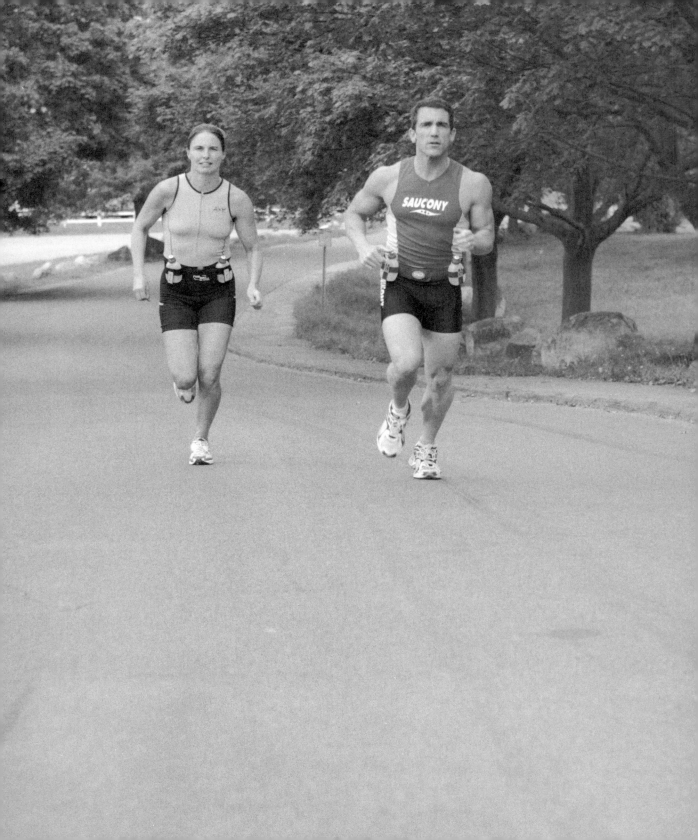

CHAPTER 1
My Coaching Philosophy

So that you may have a better understanding of my approach to triathlon training and racing, here are my main beliefs about the sport:

1. *Health comes first.* We will not sacrifice our health to achieve our sports goals. Injuries or afflictions in the name of short-term goal attainment are not acceptable. This holds true for "working through" injuries and illness; taking potentially harmful substances, both legal and illegal; undertaking training programs inappropriate for our current fitness level; and so forth. Our average life span exceeds seventy years now, and we should live those years healthy as a result of our participation in sports, not in spite of it.

2. *It's not about the bike.* To borrow the title of Lance Armstrong's book, it's not about how expensive your bike is, or that you have the top-of-the-line wetsuit, or that you keep track of your heart rate with the most advanced heart rate monitor. It's not about the gear. It's about the training, the consistency, and the balance of your work that will produce real results.

3. *Consistency is key.* When it comes to fitness, most people have an incredibly difficult time sticking with a program. Triathlon is no different, but consistency is even more crucial, because you have three different disciplines to attend to. You will get faster by simply swimming, biking, and running on a consistent basis. As Nike puts so succinctly, "Just Do It." I would add, "And Do It Often."

4. *Performance and enjoyment are not mutually exclusive.* What does this mean? Simply put, you can have fun while performing at a high level. Just because you have a scowl on your face doesn't mean that you are working really hard; conversely, if you sport a huge smile while racing, this doesn't mean that you are taking it easy. Many "old school" coaches unfortunately do not ascribe to this belief. An elite runner wrote an article in which she described running in a road race and seeing a former coach in the distance. As she called out a greeting to him, he yelled back, "If you can speak, you're not working hard enough." All I can say is that he should meet Natascha Badmann, professional female triathlete and winner of numerous Hawaii Ironman titles. She does so with a now-famous enormous smile on her face, cheering and high-fiving other competitors along the way to victory. Work hard and enjoy yourself. It's all in the mind.

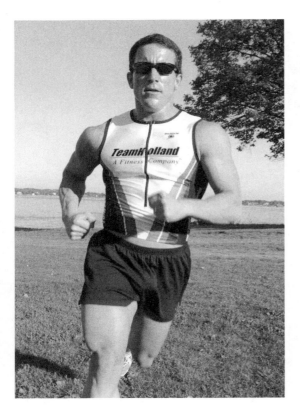

GOAL SETTING

So, you are either getting ready to attempt your first tri or you want to improve your prior performances in the sport. Either way, proper goal-setting strategies are essential to optimal performance as well as enjoyment. There are three basic goals that we can set for ourselves in sport.

Outcome goals are the ones most people set. Essentially, they involve a comparison to others or to a somewhat arbitrary value: "I will finish in the top five of my age group," or "I will do my Half-Ironman in under five hours." There are several problems with setting outcome goals as your main targets. First, quite often there is no prior race to compare it to.

This is your first time competing at the event and you choose a time based on perhaps what a friend did in his first race: "I'm more fit than he is and he did a 5:15—I can definitely beat him by a least 20 minutes." This is not an advisable goal-setting strategy. Second, there are too many uncontrollable factors that can affect your race, including the weather, equipment failures, other athletes, nutritional issues, the specific course layout, and so forth. Murphy's Law seems to play a major role in triathlon racing, so you need to be able to readjust your goals even while racing. Many pros contend that, since the race conditions are so uncontrollable in triathlon, it is the athlete who best confronts these changes that inevitably comes out on top. Last, outcome goals are black and white. You either achieve them or you fail, and this type of focus can lead to decreased enjoyment and eventual burnout.

Performance goals are a little better than outcome goals because you determine them based on a prior experience. Say you did your first sprint triathlon in 1 hour 20 minutes, then maybe for your next race you'll want to finish in 1 hour 10 minutes. You have a specific personal performance to compare it to, and this make it a little more applicable to your goal-setting strategy. This is assuming, of course, that your new time goal is "reasonable." This is where things get a little complicated. What is a "reasonable" goal? In the 1950s, most people believed that running a four-minute mile was not only impossible, but dangerous. If Roger Bannister had set a "reasonable" goal for himself, he might never have become the first person to break that barrier. So, this is where the science, training, personal inventory, and belief in one's abilities all come into play. Set your sights high, but do so with a full assessment of the total situation.

Likewise, as with outcome goals, one of the major flaws with setting performance goals is the uncontrollable conditions. Also, be careful about setting performance goals based on triathlons of the same distance but on two different courses; obviously, this disparity can drastically affect your race time.

Process goals include statements such as "I will keep my heels down during my pedal stroke," or "I will focus on having a relaxed arm swing while running," or "I will rotate my body more while swimming." These goals focus on improving a skill associated with your technique. Process goals are incredibly effective for three reasons. One, by working on and improving your process goals, inevitably your sport performance will improve and you stand to achieve both your performance and outcome goals. Two, you cannot "fail" in attaining these goals, unlike with the other two strategies. If you focus on improving your skills, you will eventually achieve positive results. Last, you can use process goals as a powerful mental tool to take your focus away from negative issues that arise during races, including pain and anxiety. Have a cramp during the run? Focus on your arm swing and you will switch your attention away from the discomfort. We will discuss this in greater detail when we look at the mental side of triathlon.

Research has indicated that the best results come from setting a combination of the three types of goals. I like to assign process goals as the primary goal(s) for myself as well as my clients; performance goals are secondary, and outcome goals come last, with the least amount of priority. A great goal for all first-time triathletes is to simply finish the race while enjoying the experience.

TRIATHLON AND MURPHY'S LAW

During my second Ironman Lake Placid, the top on my bike bottle that held my nutrition came loose as I tried to take my first drink. So, at mile 5 of the 112-mile bike ride, I was wearing 1,000 of my essential fuel calories down the front of my Saucony tri top. Needless to say, this would negatively affect my performance. Things can and will go wrong in a triathlon—it's how we learn to deal with these moments that counts. I now use bottles that screw on rather than pop open. Occasionally, for added peace of mind, I'll tape them down.

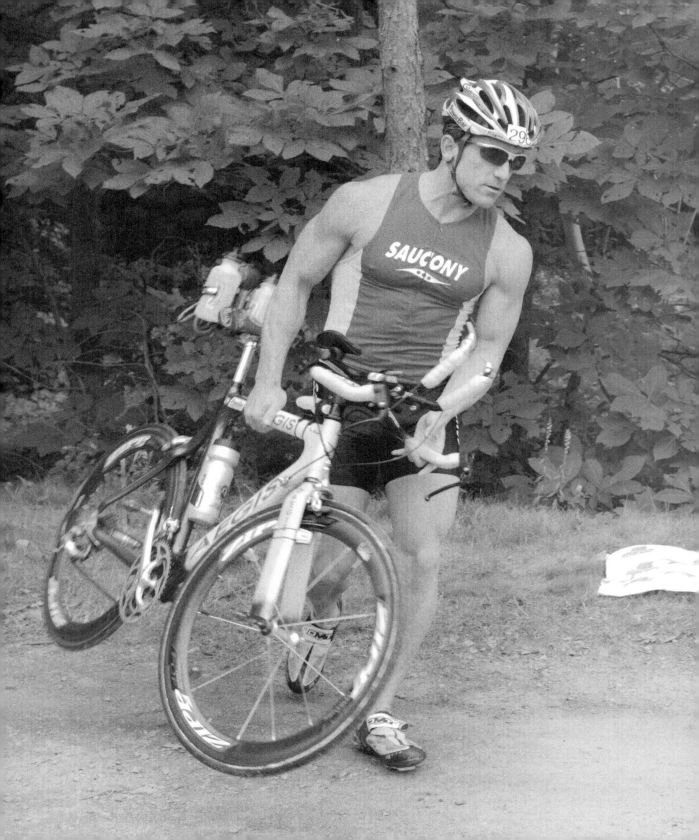

CHAPTER 2
Getting Started

THE DISTANCES

There are four basic triathlon distances, in order from shorter to longer:

1. *Sprint:* The shortest race, but also the triathlon with the most variation in distance. It is most often a .25-mile swim, 12-mile bike, and 3-mile run. Here is a list, however, of some sprint triathlons I found in the New York area held in the summer of 2004:

   - 400-yard pool swim/
     12.5-mile bike/2.9-mile run
   - 500-yard swim/12-mile bike/
     3.1-mile run
   - .25 mile-swim/15-mile bike/
     3-mile run
   - .5-mile swim/10.8-mile bike/
     3-mile run
   - .25-mile swim/11-mile bike/
     4-mile run
   - 500-yard swim/8-mile bike/
     3.1-mile run

   So, as you can see, there is quite a bit of variation in the sprint distance swim, bike, and run legs. Most of these races still take about an hour to finish, depending upon your fitness level.

2. *Olympic:* The next distance is the standard Olympic distance, which is always a 1.5-kilometer swim, 40-kilometer bike, and 10-kilometer run. This will take most people around two hours or more to complete.

3. *Half-Ironman:* This tri entails a 1.2-mile swim, 56-mile bike, and 13.1-mile run. Professional triathletes will finish these in around 4 hours, fast age-groupers will cross the finish line in around 5 hours, and most people will complete the race in 5 to 7 hours.

4. *Ironman:* A 2.4-mile swim, 112-mile bike, 26.2-mile run. There are Ironman-distance triathlons as well as specific "Ironman" tris. "Ironman" is a trade-marked term and there are only just over a dozen official Ironman triathlons worldwide. These races offer "slots" for the Ironman World Championships held every October in Kona, Hawaii. You have 17 hours to complete an Ironman to be considered an "official" finisher and receive a medal. Pros cross the line in 8 to just over 9 hours, fast age-groupers take roughly 9 to 11 hours to finish, and the rest come in after 12 to 17 hours. These races have exploded in popularity over the last few years and often fill up in less than 24 hours after registration opens. Believe it or not, there are even double and triple Ironman triathlons for those wishing to swim, bike, and run for 24 hours straight or more. These are held less frequently and have only several dozen participants, for obvious reasons.

So, which distance should you choose for your first triathlon? It makes logical sense to begin with a sprint-distance race and progress up through the distances if you wish to go longer, but this is not set in stone. Your decision will take into consideration your current level of fitness as well as the training plan you choose to follow. In other words, you can do a Half-Ironman race without ever having raced the sprint or Olympic distances if you want. If you train properly, you will have prepared yourself to go the full distance. I don't recommend doing an Ironman as your first-ever triathlon, but it can be done.

THE GEAR

Triathlon is not as simple as some sports, such as running—there is a fair amount of gear involved. And depending upon your personality type and long-term goals, your triathlon gear can become quite vast and expensive as well. For first-time triathletes or those with modest goals, the equipment need not be complicated or break the bank. Remember, it's not the machine; it's the man (or woman!) that counts. The key again is to train consistently with the

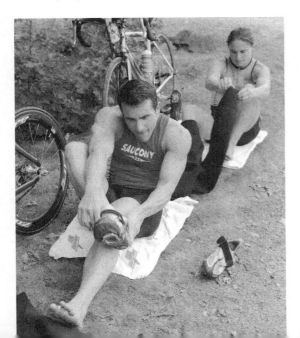

★ FINISHING TIMES

The expected finishing time for each triathlon distance depends on several factors, including your fitness level and the difficulty of the course, but rough estimates for each distance are as follows:

1. Sprint: 1–2 hours
2. Olympic: 2–3 hours
3. Half-Ironman: 4.5–6.5 hours
4. Ironman: 10–17 hours

appropriate equipment, not necessarily with the most expensive. A $10,000 bike doesn't have a motor and will not pedal for you—you still need to provide the power. As you progress in the sport and your goals become higher, then you can upgrade your equipment and add in additional training aids.

The Swim
WHAT YOU *NEED:*
   1. *A bathing suit*
   2. *Goggles*

These are the essentials for the first leg of the triathlon. There are many different types of bathing suits to choose from and many triathlon-specific suits as well. Men used to wear the infamous Speedos during the swim leg of triathlon and then often wear them on the bike and run as well. I personally am happy to see that this practice has diminished over the years. There are now several options for swimwear during triathlons; you should choose whatever you wish, depending on your personal preference:

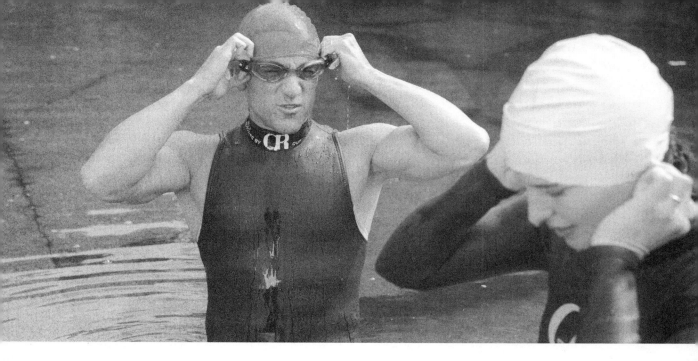

MEN:

1. *Swim trunks:* Tight-fitting, often made of spandex
2. *Tri shorts:* Similar in design to swim trunks but with additional padding for the bike segment
3. *Tri suit or skin suit:* One piece, shorts and a top, often with light padding in the seat; usually zippers down the front
4. *Tri shorts with a tri top:* Two pieces, shorts and a top, usually tight-fitting.

WOMEN:

1. *Tri suit or skin suit:* One piece, shorts and a top, often with padding.
2. *Tri shorts with a tri top:* Bikini style; two pieces, shorts and a top, usually tight-fitting.

It is your choice whether you change clothing after the swim and also after the bike.

You may wear tri shorts, a tri suit, or tri shorts with a tri top during the swim and leave it on for the rest of the race. Yes, it will be wet for part of the bike leg but the material is made to dry quickly. Just make your choice based on personal style, race goals, and comfort. Tri shorts generally do not have as much padding in them as bike shorts, so you may want to change them if you need more cushioning as you cycle. We will discuss how and where you change in the chapter on racing.

You should know that you do save a few seconds or minutes by staying in the same outfit for the entire triathlon, but often those few seconds can translate into major unpleasantness for the remainder of the race, especially the longer-distance triathlons such as the Half-Ironman and Ironman. Better to take a few extra seconds in transition and change than to suffer for hours on the bike and run.

ADDITIONAL GEAR

Wetsuit. You may need to wear a wetsuit if the water you are swimming in is very cold. It is always a good idea to check the race information about wetsuits recommendations such as "wetsuits allowed" or "wetsuits encouraged." The water is so warm in some races that wetsuits are, in fact, not allowed, but this is usually the exception. Why wear a wetsuit? Made from neoprene, wetsuits keep you warm and provide additional buoyancy, which gives you better body position in the water and therefore serves to improve your swim efficiency. Most triathletes wear a wetsuit whenever it is legal for these reasons—it makes the swim a little easier and you will have faster swim times.

So what kind should you buy? There are many different types of wetsuits on the market: sleeveless, full suits with arms, and a recently developed two-piece wetsuit with a separate bottom and top. They are not inexpensive; be prepared to pay at least $100 and around $400 for the top-of-the-line wetsuits. If you decide that you want or need a wetsuit, make sure first and foremost that it fits properly. Do not borrow one from a friend if the friend is half your size—wearing a wetsuit that is too large or too small is worse than not wearing one at all. Go to a reputable triathlon shop and get fitted correctly. Do not buy a wetsuit over the Internet if you are not absolutely sure that it is the correct size for you. Purchase one based on your goals and your budget. It will last a long time if you take proper care of it. Like an expensive bike, however, an expensive wetsuit will improve your performance, but only to a point. If do not practice your swim, a wetsuit will really only keep you warmer and closer to the water's surface while you swim poorly.

Swim cap. A swim cap is more important for men and women with long hair, to keep it tucked away in the water. Most races will give you one in your race packet, and quite often it will be color-coded according to your age group. Regardless of your hair length, it is a good idea to get used to wearing one during training as you might be required to wear one in your race.

The Bike
WHAT YOU *NEED*:
1. *A bike*
2. *A helmet*

As I stated before, I did my first few triathlons on a rented bike and rented helmet. My brother Dan did his first race, an Olympic distance tri, on a beat-up mountain bike. The bike is obviously the most expensive piece of equipment involved in triathlon. As the race distance

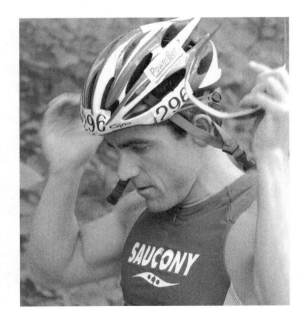

increases and your goals become loftier, the more important the quality of the bike becomes. What I have come to realize about triathlon is that many people enjoy "dressing" the part—it is most definitely a sport where if you invest enough money, you can really look like a pro. A custom bike, race wheels, fancy jersey, colorful helmet, cool shades, and so on. I have a friend who bought an incredibly expensive bike, yet he refuses to ride it in the rain, get it dirty, so he rarely rides it at all. I think he must just clean it constantly and admire it in his basement. I think he might even wrap it in plastic, like some people do to protect their furniture. What's my point? You need not invest in an extremely expensive bike to participate in triathlon. Beginners at the sprint and Olympic distance can pretty much ride anything with two wheels to start. So, if your goal is just to finish a shorter-distance tri, you can use your mountain bike or your hybrid and you will do fine.

Those participating in the Half-Ironman- and Ironman-distance tris will need a bike more suited for those longer distances. There are two basic types of bikes to choose from, road bikes and triathlon bikes. What's the difference? There are primarily two:

Geometry: A triathlon-specific bike has what is known as a more "aggressive" geometry as far as the seat tube angle is concerned. It is designed as such to put the rider in a more "aerodynamic" position. This advantage does sacrifice some comfort and takes some getting used to.

"Aero" Bars: These are special handlebars that also put the rider in a more aerodynamic position. One of the major forces that the biker is working against is wind resistance, so any advantage in this area will translate into faster race times. Once again, comfort is sacrificed for this speed advantage and riding in the aero position requires practice as well as core strength and flexibility. There are clip-on aerobars that can be mounted right on your regular road bike and aerobars that are connected directly to the bicycle and cannot be removed.

Do you need a triathlon-specific bike and aerobars? If you have goals that are more than just simply finishing, or, most importantly, if you are willing to invest the money, then by all means, buy a nice tri bike. It's an investment in your health and will last a long time if you take care of it. Be prepared to pay roughly $1,000 for an entry-level bike and $3,000 to $5,000 for a higher-end model.

PEDALS

While the bicycles we rode as kids had flat pedals, road bikes and tri bikes are a little more advanced. Most come with one of the following two setups for pedals:

Cages: Exactly as they sound, these pedals have "cages" that you slide your running shoes into. They are more efficient than basic flat pedals as they allow you to pull up on the pedals and transfer power more effectively.

Clipless: More advanced than simple cages, these pedals require special bike shoes that clip into the pedals themselves. This design offers the most efficient method of pedaling. There are several different types of clipless pedal systems to choose from and many triathletes choose theirs based on personal preference.

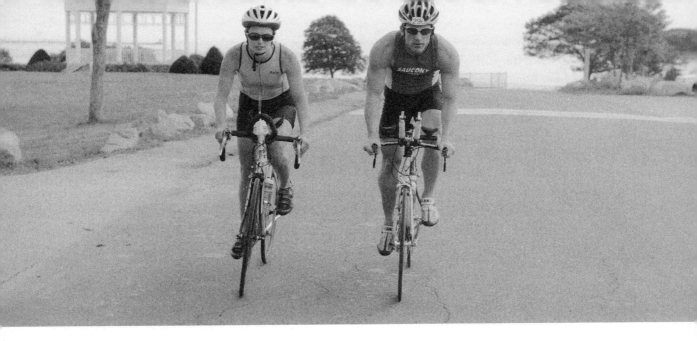

WHEELS

Bikes come with two sizes of wheels: 650 and 700. Smaller riders will generally ride 650s while taller bikers will use 700s. The bike specialist will choose the appropriate size for you when you are purchasing your bike.

There are also two types of tires to choose from on your wheels: clinchers and tubulars.

Clinchers are the more common type of tire used as they are much less expensive than tubulars and many find them a little easier to change. There are two pieces involved, the tire itself and the tube. The tube goes inside the tire, and when you get a flat, you simply pull out the damaged tube and replace it with a new one. The whole process takes only a few minutes once you become adept at performing the change.

Tubulars, also known as "sew ups," are much more expensive than clincher tubes. Tubulars are just one piece; the tire and the tube are not separate. These tires need to be "glued" onto the wheel rim, which is another reason why many prefer clinchers over tubulars. When you flat with a tubular, you need to break the seal of the glue and pull the entire tire off of the wheel rim. You then place a new tubular tire on the rim, one that has been "preglued," which means it has dried glue on it already. The glue on the tire and the glue that is already on the wheel rim combine to secure the new tire in place. You simply inflate it and you are ready to go. Some people use both clinchers and tubulars; they will use clinchers on their "training wheels" and tubulars on their race wheels. This way they save money by replacing only the more inexpensive tubes with the clinchers during training and use the tubulars during the race—tubulars are less likely to flat and many find that, with practice, they can change the one-piece tubulars a little faster during a race.

I use the clincher-during-training and tubular-while-racing strategy myself. If your goal is performance based and you have money to spend, then you can choose to have two sets of wheels (or more!).

Training wheels. These relatively inexpensive wheels are made for durability and not necessarily speed. They are generally heavier than race rims and can withstand the rigors of heavy training over a variety of road surfaces.

Race wheels. Your expensive superlight wheels. These you ride sparingly during training and save for race day.

Disc wheels. These are solid wheels that do not have spokes. This increased surface area is more aerodynamic than wheels with spokes and therefore will translate into slightly faster race times as a result of their use. They are used as your back wheel. Generally more expensive than your average wheel, they are primarily used on flat courses where there is low wind. When used on windy courses, the disc wheel can act like a sail and be difficult to control. Again, if performance is your goal, you have extra money to burn, and you intend on riding on somewhat flat courses with low wind, then you can consider having a disc wheel as an option on race day.

ADDITIONAL GEAR

Bike shoes. If you use clips for pedals, you will need specific bike shoes. These vary greatly in price and design, and you should select yours based on your goals and budget.

Bike gloves. Often fingerless and padded, bike gloves may be used to provide added comfort as well as protection in the event of a fall.

Bike shorts. Try riding for any amount of time in regular shorts and you will soon realize the necessity for bike shorts. They are tight to decrease chafing and padded to lessen the discomfort, especially during longer rides. Invest in a quality bike short—the additional expense is well worth it.

Bike jersey. Tight-fitting, with sleeves or without, often quite colorful and covered with foreign terms and product logos that will make you feel like a sponsored athlete. I recommend choosing bright colors so that you are highly visible to motorists during your training on the roads.

Sunglasses. A mixture of fashion and function. They are recommended not only for protection from the sun, but for picking up significant speed during your bike rides, especially on downhills. Taking a bug in the eye at 40 miles an hour or more can be an unpleasant experience to say the least.

Trip computer. From the inexpensive and simple to pricey and very technologically advanced, bike computers can measure speed, average speed, distance, ride time, cadence, power, and even your heart rate. This data can even be downloaded directly to your computer for record-keeping and analysis. They come with or without cords, and they mount on your handlebars. It tracks your wheel rotation via magnet (attached to one of your bike spokes) and a sensor on your fork.

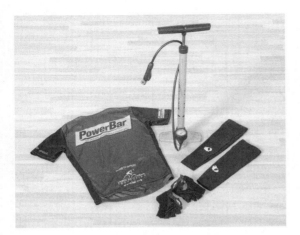

Pictured clockwise: Floor pump, arm warmers, bike gloves, bike jersey

Bike pump. To inflate your tires. There are floor pumps that show inflation level to use before races and smaller pumps to bring with you during training rides.

Multipurpose bike tool. To tighten screws and make small adjustments when necessary.

Tire levers. Small tools that you use when you change your tires.

Bike bag. A bag that attaches to your frame to hold items during rides, including spare tubes, your bike tool, tire levers, et cetera.

Spare tubes or tubulars. Spare tubes if you are using wheels with clinchers or spare tubulars if you choose that type of wheel.

PURCHASING YOUR FIRST BIKE

So, you have decided to jump right in and purchase your first tri bike. When choosing a bike shop, try to find one that:

1. *Comes recommended by others.*
2. *Has employees who are familiar with triathlon.* There is a difference between the sports of cycling and triathlon; ideally, you want to work with someone who understands the nuances between the two.
3. *Knows how to correctly "fit" you to your new bike.* This is crucial. Again, you will really only know this by feedback from others who have bought bikes there and were pleased with their bike fit. When shopping for your bike, ask the bike shop employee how long the bike fit process takes—it should realistically take at least an hour to get you in a comfortable and biomechanically correct position. You may encounter the situation where you find a great deal on a bike at a local shop, the bike having the correct size frame, but the employees are not trained to fit you into the proper triathlon position. In this case, you can buy the bike and then get it fitted elsewhere.

WHEN CHOOSING A BIKE

Let's be totally honest—many people base their bike purchase on the same simple criteria that they would employ in choosing a car or making any other major purchase:

1. *Brand:* The cool people have one.
2. *Looks:* I, too, will look cool on it. I personally always wanted a Softride bike, not for any other reason than I thought it looked great because of the unique suspension bar holding up the seat.

As you can see in the sidebar describing the bikes ridden at the Hawaii World Championships, there are more than twenty brands

WHAT BRAND OF BIKE SHOULD I BUY?

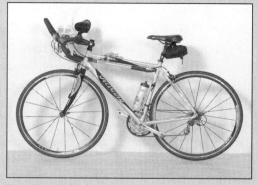

#10. Specilaized-34

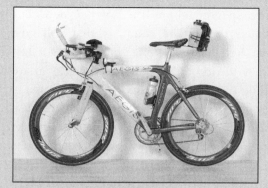

#14. Aegis-20 (Tom's bike)

I often say if you want to know what to do when it comes to sports, look at what the professionals are doing. The following is a breakdown of the bikes represented at the 2002 Ironman Hawaii World Championships, ridden by the some of the best 1,500 triathletes in the world. Many of these brands have bikes that run from the relatively inexpensive models up to the extremely expensive.

1. Kestrel-156
2. Trek-143
3. Cannondale-139
4. Litespeed-94
5. Quintana Roo-70
6. Softride-69
7. Cervelo-57
8. Principia-48
9. Griffen-46
10. Specialized-34
11. Giant-32
12. Felt-21
13. Look-21
14. Aegis-20
15. Calfee-18
16. Colnago-18
17. Cube-18
18. Klein-16
19. Merlin-13
20. Serotta-12
21. Bianchi-11
22. Storck-11
23. Corima-9
24. GT-8

represented. It is also worth noting that the professional triathletes will often change bike brands from year to year, not because of anything specific about the bike design, but because that is the company that will give them free bikes and pay them sponsorship money to ride them. Start with what you are willing to spend and stick to it. The frame is the most important first investment because you can upgrade the other elements, such as the components, seat, wheels, et cetera, later as you wish. I believe that you can buy a decent new entry-level triathlon bike for $800 to $1,200, less if you find one used. If money is no object, than feel free to drop $5,000 on that LiteSpeed with the Zipp racing wheels. Just realize that if you do buy the top-of-the-line bike, you can't blame the equipment for a poor race performance!

BIKE FIT

There unfortunately exists an inverse relationship between comfort and aerodynamics when it comes to bike fit. Remember, you need to run after your bike leg, and if you have been riding in an uncomfortable position, it will greatly affect your run performance. This is especially important when competing in half- and full Ironman triathlons. So, consider comfort first, and aerodynamic body position second. Five minutes saved through reduced wind resistance while biking in an extreme aero position can translate into a stiff back for the run, which could ultimately slow your run by much more than five minutes. It can also lead to injury over time.

We each have a unique body; therefore, someone else's aero position might not be correct for you. We each have an individual

BUYING A BIKE ON THE INTERNET

You may know the exact bike you want, size and all, and may want to purchase it on the Internet at such Web sites as eBay. You can indeed find incredible bargains on bikes as well as all kinds of triathlon gear using this method. Again, many triathletes are forever upgrading and therefore are often willing to part with their old gear at drastically reduced prices. If you choose to buy a bike over the Internet, be sure that you know your correct frame size and have it fitted for you by a qualified technician.

STICK WITH WHAT WORKS

Many years ago I went into my favorite running store, Super Runner's Shop, in New York City to purchase a new pair of running shoes. I frequent and recommend this store because the employees are all runners themselves, and they are all incredibly knowledgeable about their sport. When I informed the salesman that I needed a new pair, he looked down at my feet and said, "A new pair of Saucony 3D Grid Hurricanes?" No, I replied, I wanted to try a new brand. "Did you have a problem with these?" he asked. No, I replied again, I just wanted something new. "If they work for you, then you stick with them." Incredibly wise words, and I have used Saucony 3D Grid Hurricanes ever since. There are just so many variables in sport when it comes to performance and injury that, when you know definitively that something works, you do not change it.

biomechanical makeup, different levels of flexibility, and so on that determine our own best riding position. Because Tim DeBoom rides a certain way does not mean that is what you should do. Over your tri career, you will constantly make slight changes to your bike setup in an attempt to find the ideal riding position for you. These are the primary places you will adjust your bike fit:

1. *Seat height*
2. *Seat position fore/aft*
3. *Handlebar height*
4. *Aerobar pad spacing*
5. *Aerobar length*
   (if you have an adjustable model)

Again, have a qualified bike mechanic set these initial positions for you. Over time, you can make minor adjustments as you feel may be necessary. Always remember that comfort comes first.

The Run
WHAT YOU *NEED*:
   1. *Running shoes*

That's what's so great about running; all you need are a pair of shoes and you are good to go. Of course, you'll want to have running clothes as well, but proper footwear is the only essential equipment. Many people ask me to recommend the "best" brand of running shoes, and my reply is "What works best for you." There is no "best" pair of running shoes per se. Everyone has unique biomechanics, such as type of arches, pronation versus supination, foot width, and weekly mileage that respond to specific shoe designs. I have "fat feet," wide at the toebox, and Saucony makes a line of shoes that have worked great for me over the years. This leads me to the number one rule of choosing your running shoe:

It's about function, not fashion.

The ugliest running shoe may be the one that is perfect for you—that's the one you need. Buying a shoe just because it looks great may lead to injury down the road. The wrong shoe can do just that, cause injuries to the feet, knees, and hips.

BUYING RUNNING SHOES

Once again, you want to buy your shoes in a specialty running store, if possible. Ideally, the salesperson will be a runner himself and will ask you questions, including how many miles a week you run, how long you have been running, if you race, and if you do race, what distances. They should look at your current pair of running shoes to observe the wear patterns on the soles; this can help them determine your individual patterns of pronation and supination. He should also watch you run a short distance to observe your gait, how your feet strike the ground. More advanced stores now have treadmills in them so that the running shoe specialist can observe and even videotape the customer's running style to aid in the shoe selection process.

Beware of purchasing running shoes in a store that sells much more than running gear and apparel. If you are surrounded by such items as camping gear, fishing poles, and guns as you are selecting your running shoes, odds are you may not end up with what you need.

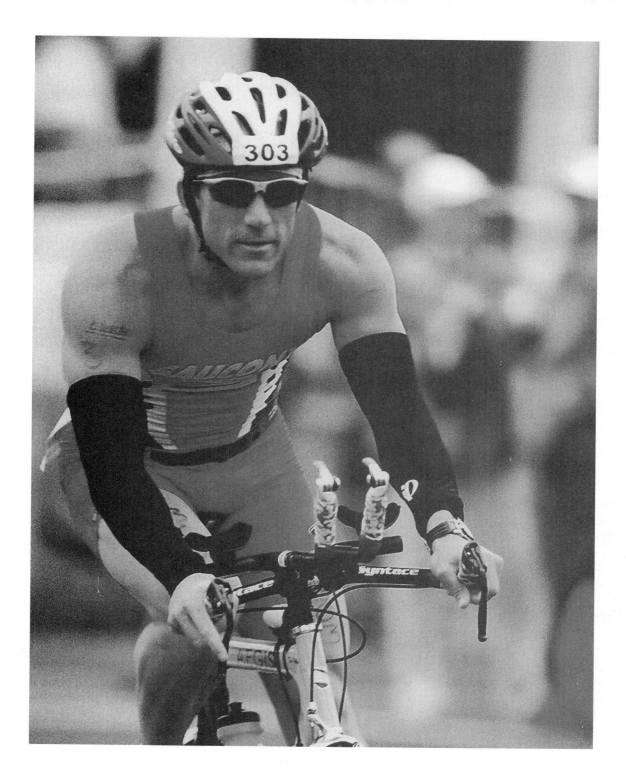

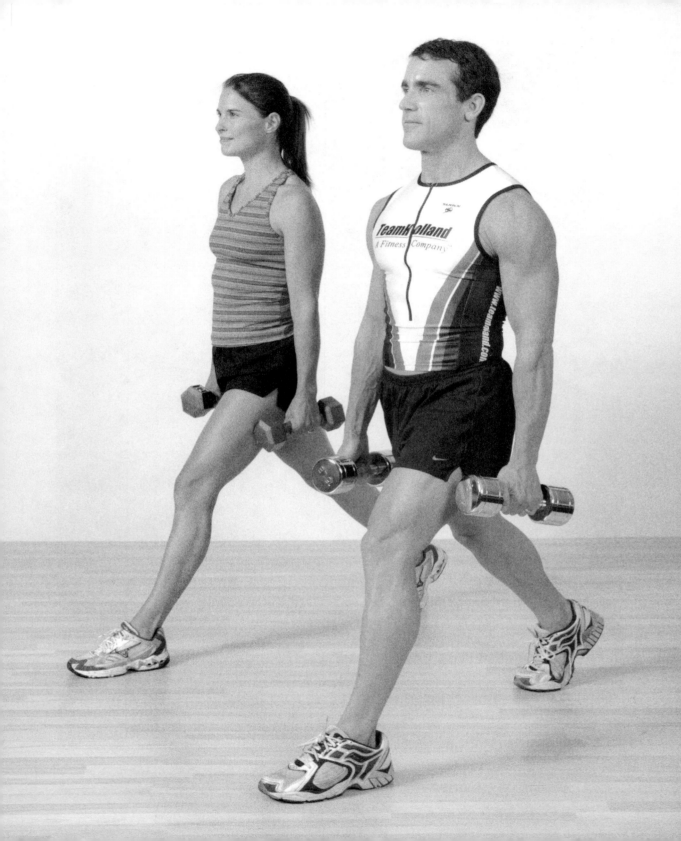

CHAPTER 3
Strength Training

If you have skipped ahead and read the training plans, you may have noticed that all eight of them contain two weight training sessions per week up until the Taper Phase, when we pull out the strength work. You may wonder why you should "waste" two sessions per week on strength training instead of spending that time either swimming, biking, or running. This is a triathlon training program, not a bodybuilding contest, right? Absolutely right.

It was not too long ago that runners, cyclists, and triathletes all avoided lifting weights. It simply was not done. These athletes believed that building muscle would be incredibly detrimental to their performances. Lifting weights would cause a person to become "muscle-bound"; flexibility would be lost and race times would become slower. The prevailing belief was, if you want to become better at your sport, then you should simply practice that sport as much as possible. This thinking has changed dramatically over the past decade as current research has proven all of these myths to be false. This is not to say that it is okay to lift like a bodybuilder; each sport has its own specific resistance training designs and protocols. And this field is relatively new; many coaches have dramatically different approaches to strength training as it applies to their athletes.

What I have found in my studies and through coaching hundreds of athletes is that strength training does, in fact, serve three primary purposes for athletes in general and triathletes specifically. It:

1. *Corrects individual biomechanical issues*
2. *Prevents injury*
3. *Improves performance*

And these are in order of importance, in my personal opinion.

CORRECTING INDIVIDUAL BIOMECHANICAL ISSUES

So what does "correcting individual biomechanical issues" mean exactly? Well, I have met hundreds upon hundreds of people who tell me that they would love to run or do a triathlon but they can't because they have "bad knees." What are "bad knees"? So often this condition is the result of individual biomechanical issues, not the least of which are muscle issues that can be dealt with through strength training. Weak leg extensor muscles can lead to improper tracking of your kneecap (patella), which can lead to "bad knees." An imbalance between your hamstring strength and quadriceps strength can also lead to knee pain. This type of imbalance is common in many athletes who participate in one sport exclusively, such as running; they create strength imbalances that will ultimately lead to injury. This is why strength training is so crucial when it comes to sports such as triathlon. I often say it is not the sport that causes the injury per se, it only illuminates "weak links" and where changes need to be made. "Shin splints," pain in the front of the lower leg, a common injury in runners, is quite often caused by doing "too much too soon" but can also be the result of weak calf muscles (gastrocnemius and soleus muscles), weak muscles in the shin (anterior tibialis), or a strength imbalance between the two. The analogy of a chain applies to the body and sports; you are only as strong as your weakest link. Also, the place on your body where the pain presents itself is quite often the symptom of a biomechanical issue elsewhere. A weakness in one hip muscle, for example, can change your gait, forcing you to improperly modify your stride, and thus create pain in another muscle, such as one hamstring. This is why doctors cannot easily diagnose sports-related injuries right away; it is often an investigative process of sorts that takes time to uncover the underlying issues. The bottom line is that you need to strength train, engage in full-body workouts, creating a strong, balanced body that will only get stronger through triathlon training, not break down as a result of it.

PREVENTING INJURY

Many triathletes would say that they don't strength train because they don't have the time. Their reasoning is that, given a limited amount of time to train for three separate sports, strength training is simply not that important in the grand scheme of things. Why waste time in the gym when the race involves swimming, biking, and running?

Unfortunately, quite often these are the people who end up in physical therapy with "bad knees" and "bad backs." No matter how disciplined you are with your triathlon training, if you are injured, you will eventually be forced

FIXING THE WEAK LINKS

I had a client who wanted to begin a running program but had been experiencing major back pain for some time. She was seeing a chiropractor three times a week for adjustments just to minimize her daily pain. I brought her to the gym to test her overall strength and found that she had incredible muscle weakness in the lower body, so much so that she could barely perform one repetition of certain exercises with almost no weight. We focused on strengthening these imbalances, and before long, she had ceased the chiropractic adjustments and completed her first half-marathon.

to scale back or cease training altogether. You must consider strength training to be an essential component of your overall program. This is especially true during the first four weeks of your training, the Base Phase. Think of it as if you were building a house; the first and most important step is to lay down a solid foundation. If you skip or rush through this step, the house will be weak and eventually present structural problems. Strength training is not a choice but a necessity when it comes to participation in sport.

Again, just as strength training serves to correct individual biomechanical issues, which prevents injuries, it likewise strengthens weaknesses and corrects imbalances that arise as a result of training, also preventing injury. I meet many older runners who ran years ago, many miles per week, and now say that they can no longer run because they have some injury as a result. Running was their primary exercise and they did not lift weights. I would argue that more often than not, it is the participation in one endeavor exclusively that causes problems, not the endeavor itself. Anything done to extremes is bound to eventually cause problems. Run eighty miles a week and nothing else? Chances are you will experience problems. Swim three hours a day exclusively? I can bet you will experience injury, and I'd put my money on it arising at the shoulder complex. The more you participate in a sport, the more crucial it is to engage in strength training to prevent injury. Recent research has indicated that running is, in fact, not necessarily bad for your knees. In an examination of runners who had been running for many years, it was found that they had no higher incidence of such issues as arthritis. In fact, two of the worst things you can do for your knee joints are not to be active and to carry around excessive amounts of weight. Running and participation in triathlon training will help with both of these issues, and strength training will allow you to do both for many years to come. And the strength training encompasses your entire body, not just your legs. When you run, you do not leave your upper body at home—it is involved as well! Upper body, lower back, abdominal muscles, and all the major muscles of the lower body must be strengthened and balanced to keep you injury-free and enjoying triathlon for many years to come.

IMPROVING PERFORMANCE

The scientific and anecdotal evidence both indicate that strength training does, in fact, improve performance when it comes to swimming, biking, and running. In other words, studies in the laboratory as well as observations made by real people and professional athletes alike point to the incredible performance benefits of strength training. Lift weights and you will indeed go faster and longer! Mark Allen, six-time Hawaii Ironman winner and now triathlon coach is a strong advocate of strength training for triathletes. Pick any sport and you would be hard pressed to find an athlete who excels in that sport who does not engage in some form of weight training. The key is to lift weights appropriately for your sport; for us, triathlon. The strength training program we engage in as triathletes is markedly different from the program that, say, a football player would follow. In fact, resistance training has evolved to the point that it is so highly specific that players within a certain sport will not necessarily follow the same strength training program. A running back in football will not have the same routine that his fellow linemen will follow. A great resistance training program is not merely thrown together. It takes into account the specific demands of the sport and the motor pattern involved. It utilizes the appropriate exercise selection, load (weight), sets, repetitions, rest intervals, sequencing, and periodization. It is both a science and an art. We can train our bodies for increased strength, power, and endurance—all really important factors in our triathlon performances.

MORE ABOUT WHY STRENGTH TRAINING IS IMPORTANT

A perceived lack of time is the major reason many people give for not lifting weights. (I say "perceived" because I believe it is a choice; we find time to do the things we wish to do. Just look at how long people will wait in line to get an ice cream cone.) The other three major reasons people avoid strength training are:

1. They don't know what to do.
2. They worry about injuring themselves.
3. They don't have the necessary equipment.

As for not knowing what to do, I have provided a triathlon-specific strength training program for you to follow. I'll tell you exactly what to do and how often to do it. It entails a total-body workout, the primary focus of which is to build a strong base of strength. This will, in turn, improve your imbalances and weaknesses, improving your triathlon performance while minimizing your chances of injury. It is relatively simple and is not time-consuming; the key is to do it consistently.

When people do injure themselves while weight training, it's usually because they perform the exercises incorrectly and/or with an excessive amount of weight. I designed this twelve-week strength training program with detailed descriptions on proper form for each exercise. Again, you don't have to perform complex exercises to accomplish your strength training goals. You also don't have to use great amounts of weight, either. The guideline for how much weight you should use is this: the last few repetitions of each exercise should be difficult, but you can still maintain proper form. This is crucial—use weights that are too light, and you will not get the results you seek; use weights that are too heavy, and you will potentially injure yourself. Always pay strict attention to your form and stop the exercise if your form is compromised.

Are you worried about not having a gym membership or that your gym has a limited selection of machines? No problem. The strength training program I designed uses a minimal amount of equipment, and you can do it in the privacy of your home. Don't misunderstand, "minimal equipment" doesn't mean that the program is any less effective—in fact, the most effective exercises require no equipment at all. A stability ball, dumbbells, and a mat are all that you will need for this strength training program. These are all relatively inexpensive, and you should be able to purchase everything for under fifty dollars.

Things to Think about While Strength Training

1. *Form.* Again, good form is crucial when lifting weights, not only to prevent injury, but also to achieve your desired results.

I cannot stress this point enough. I can't tell you the percentage of people I see working who have incredibly poor form. Pay close attention to the description of each exercise and use mirrors if possible to see your what you look like so you can make corrections when necessary. When your form fails, it is time to end the exercise.

2. *Tempo.* This refers to the speed at which you perform each individual repetition. Most people do this too fast, which is no surprise, because that makes the workout easier! For our purposes, we will adhere to a two-second/four-second rule. This essentially means that we will lower the weight (or our body) a little more slowly than we raise it. For example, if you are doing a biceps curl, you would take two seconds to bring the weight up toward your shoulder, then take four seconds to lower it back to the starting position. If you are performing a stationary squat, you would lower your body on a four count, then come back up on a count of two. Sounds simple, but it isn't, and very few people do exercises in this manner. The four-count is very important: most people lose the down phase of each exercise, and this is one major reason why they don't see results. You lose one of the most crucial parts of the exercise when you allow gravity or momentum to do the work for you. When in doubt, slow it down.

3. *Appropriate weight.* Quite simply put, men generally lift weights that are too heavy, whereas women lift weights that are too light. Both lead to diminished results. The rule of thumb is that you want to use a weight where the last few repetitions are difficult, yet you can complete them with good form. When the last few repetitions become too easy, then it is time to increase the weight.

4. *Rest intervals.* You shouldn't really spend more than an hour strength training if you do it efficiently, and each session should truly be much shorter, even full-body workouts. Most of us waste time between exercises. When training for endurance and basic strength, thirty to sixty seconds is all the time you should rest in between sets. There is a physiological reason for this along with simply keeping your workout time down to a minimum. By taking short rest intervals, you are not allowing your muscles to fully recover. This trains the endurance component of your muscles while building strength at the same time, something we as triathletes are looking to achieve. True power lifters will take three to five minutes in between sets to allow their bodies to recover completely so that they can lift as much as possible on the next attempt. Our goals are different, which is good; this means that we want to keep our rest to a minimum, which makes our workouts shorter.

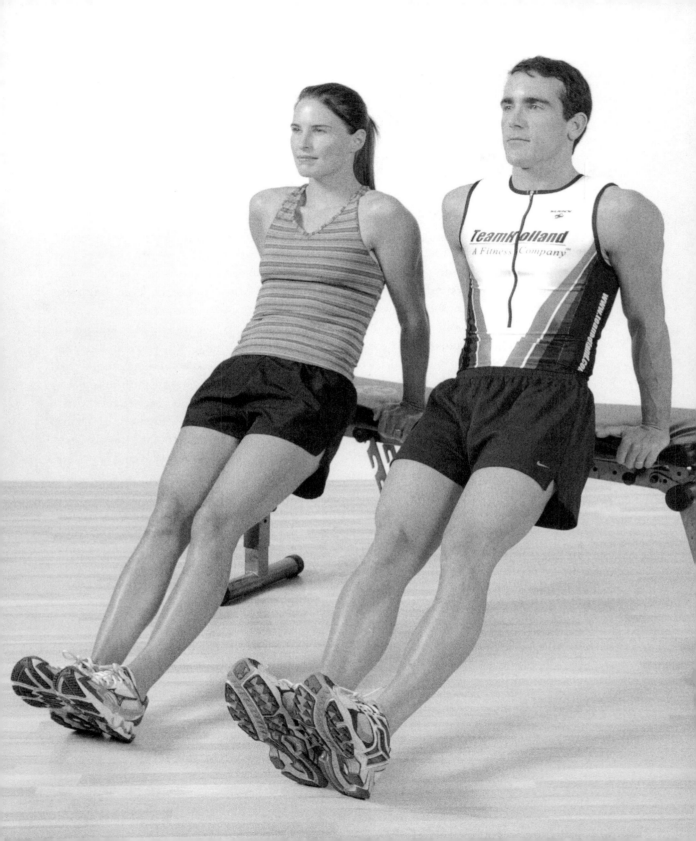

CHAPTER 4

Triathlon Resistance Training Program

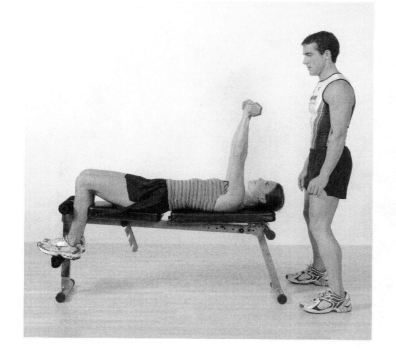

BASE TRAINING PHASE

Dumbbell Chest Presses
Muscle focus: Chest
Sets: 2
Reps: 12

Lie on a flat bench holding dumbbells with your arms bent to 90 degrees and your elbows level with your shoulders. Press the weights up and over your chest until the ends are almost touching, then lower back down.

Dumbbell Bent-Over Rows
Muscle focus: Back
Sets: 2
Reps: 12

Place one arm and one knee on a bench for balance while holding a dumbbell in the other hand. Position your upper body so that it is parallel to the floor and the natural curve remains in your lower back. Begin with your arm extended down toward the floor; then raise the weight up toward your armpit. Hold for one second, then lower.

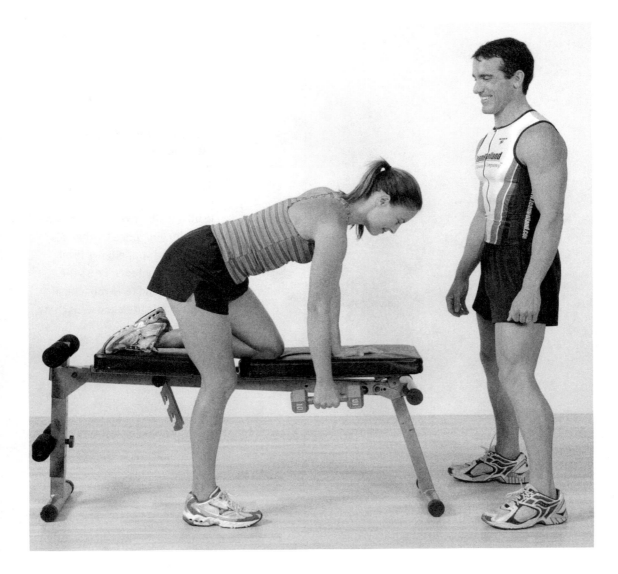

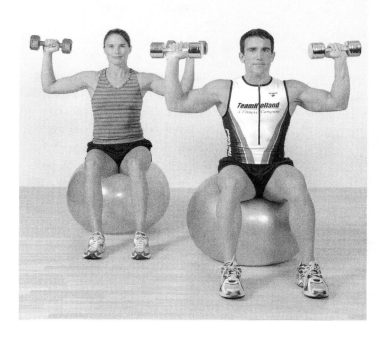

Dumbbell Overhead Presses
Muscle focus: Shoulders
Sets: 2
Reps: 12

This may be done while sitting or standing. Hold dumbbells up with your elbows in line with your shoulders and your palms facing forward. Press them over your head until the ends are almost touching, then slowly lower them back down to the starting position.

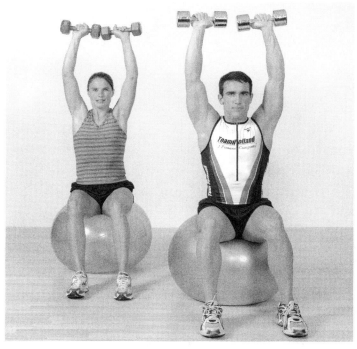

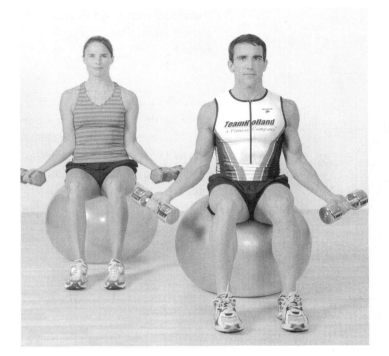

Dumbbell Biceps Curls
Muscle focus: Biceps
Sets: 2
Reps: 12

You can do this sitting or standing. Hold the dumbbells with your elbows tucked into your sides and your palms facing forward. Slowly raise the weights toward your shoulders. Hold for one second, then slowly lower down.

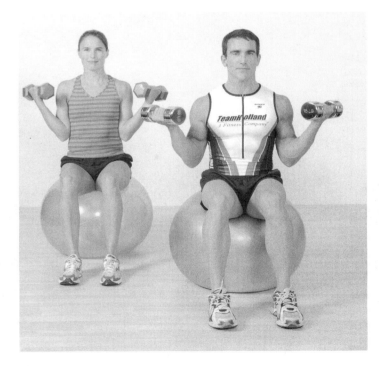

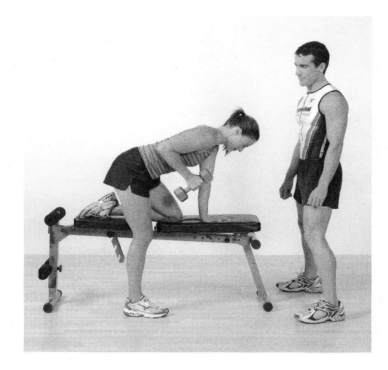

Dumbbell Kick Backs
Muscle focus: Triceps
Sets: 2
Reps: 12

Place one arm and one knee on a bench for balance while holding a dumbbell in the other hand. Position your upper body so that it is parallel to the floor and bring your elbow up so that your upper arm is parallel to the floor as well. With your palm facing toward you, lift the weight back and up until your arm is fully extended, hold for one second, then slowly lower back down. Keep your upper arm stable throughout the exercise.

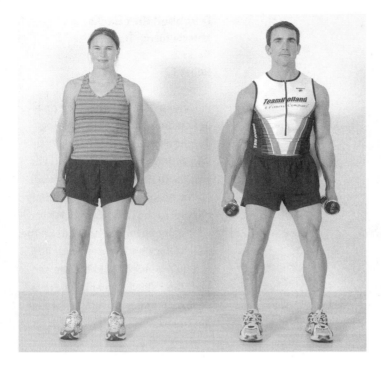

Stability Ball Squats
(dumbbells optional)

Muscle focus: Glutes, hamstrings, quadriceps

Sets: 2

Reps: 12

Stand while pressing a stability ball into a wall with your back. Your feet should be a little wider than shoulder width apart, with your toes pointing forward. Keeping your chest up and knees behind your toes, lower your body down to just above 90 degrees of knee bend, hold for one second, then return to starting position.

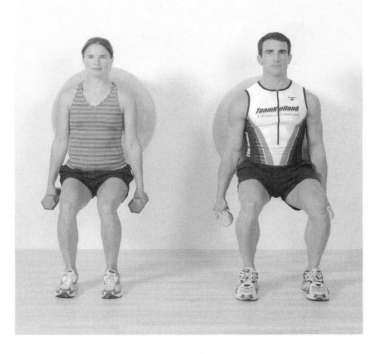

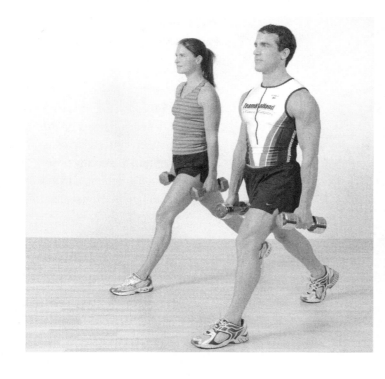

Stationary Lunges
(dumbbells optional)
Muscle focus: Glutes, hamstrings, quadriceps
Sets: 2
Reps: 12 both legs

Stand in a split stance with one leg forward and one back. Making sure to keep your chest up and your knee behind your toes, lower your body straight down to the floor until your back knee is almost touching the floor. Hold for one second, then return to starting position.

Stability Ball Hamstring Curls

Muscle focus: Hamstrings
Sets: 2
Reps: 12

Lie on your back on the floor with your hips raised and heels on the stability ball. Pull the ball to your butt, then return to starting position. Do not allow your hips to touch the floor throughout the exercise.

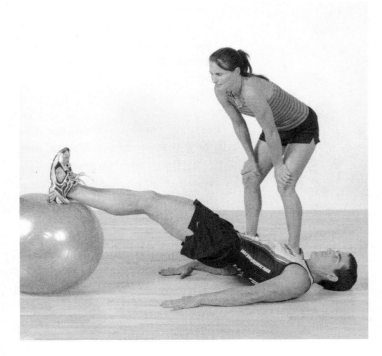

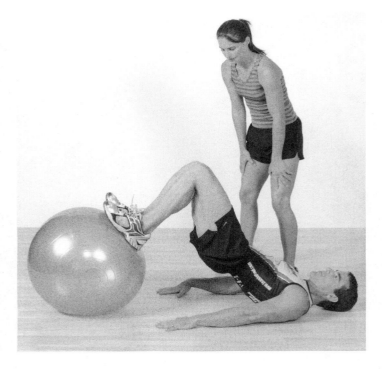

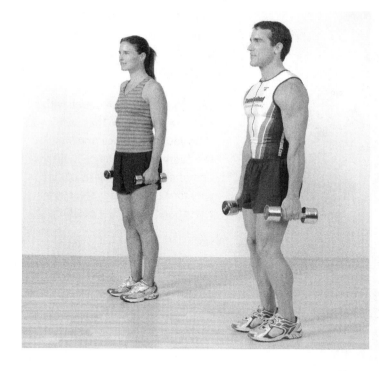

Calf Raises
(dumbbells optional)
Muscles focus: Calves
Sets: 2
Reps: 12

Stand with feet shoulder-width apart. Raise your body up in the air and your heels off of the ground by pressing down on your toes, then lower back down to starting position.

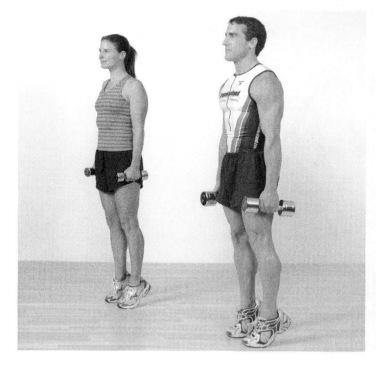

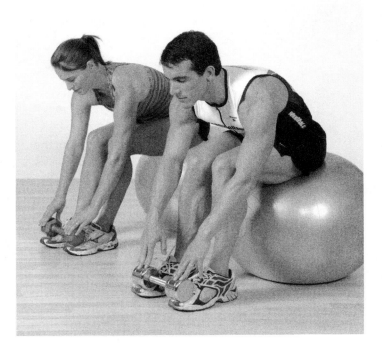

Dumbbell Toe Raises
Muscle focus: Shins
Sets: 2
Reps: 12

Sit on a chair, bench or ball with a dumbbell placed so that each end is on your toes. Place one hand on the dumbbell to balance it, lift the dumbbell up in the air by curling your toes toward your shins, then lower back to starting position.

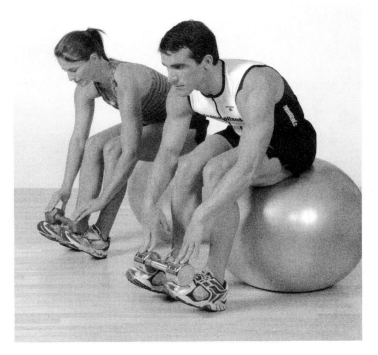

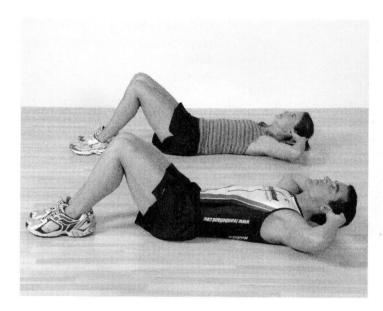

Regular Crunches
Muscle focus: Abs
Sets: 1
Reps: 25

Lie on the floor with your knees bent and your hands behind your head. Keeping your chin off of your chest, slowly lift your upper body up off the floor, hold for one second, then lower back down.

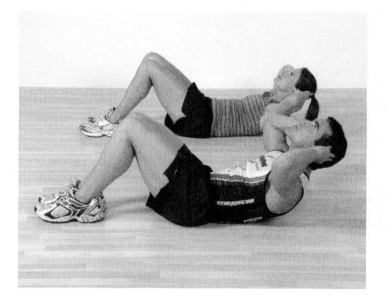

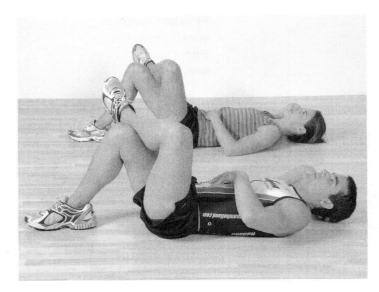

Oblique Twists

Muscle focus: Abs (obliques)
Sets: 1
Reps: 25 each side

Lie on the floor with one knee bent and the other leg crossed with the ankle resting on the thigh. Place your opposite hand of the leg that is raised behind your head, then bring that elbow toward your raised foot while twisting and bringing that shoulder blade up off the floor. Lower back down but do not allow the shoulder blade to touch the floor for the remainder of the exercise.

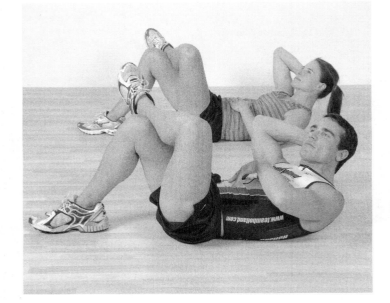

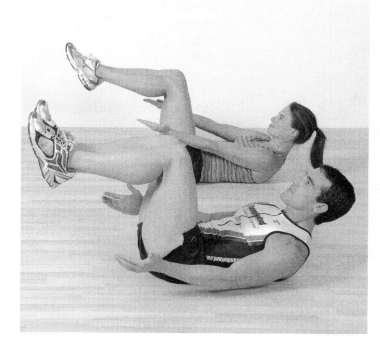

Reverse Crunches
Muscle focus: Abs (lower)
Sets: 1
Reps: 25

Lie on your back with your feet raised in the air with 90 degrees of knee bend and your lower back pressed firmly into the floor. Making sure to keep the lower back firmly down, reach away from your body with your feet until your legs are almost fully extended, hold for one second, then return to starting position.

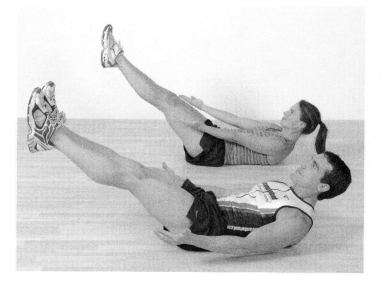

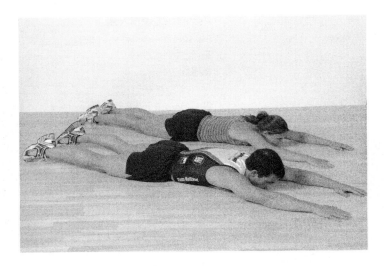

Superman

Muscle focus: Spinal erectors
Sets: 1
Reps: 10

Lie on you stomach with your arms straight above your head. Simultaneously lift both hands and feet up off the floor, squeezing the muscles of your lower back; hold for one second, then slowly lower back down.

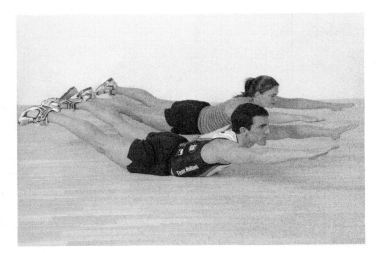

Plank

Muscle focus: Abdominals and lower back
Sets: 1
Reps: 1 minute

Assume a push-up position but support your upper body with your forearms and your palms pressed together. Keep your body perfectly straight and your abdominals tight, and breathe normally. Hold this position for one minute or until you lose your form. At the beginning, if your form fails early, then you may rest on your knees for a few seconds, then return to plank position and hold, repeating this for one minute. The goal is to hold for one minute straight.

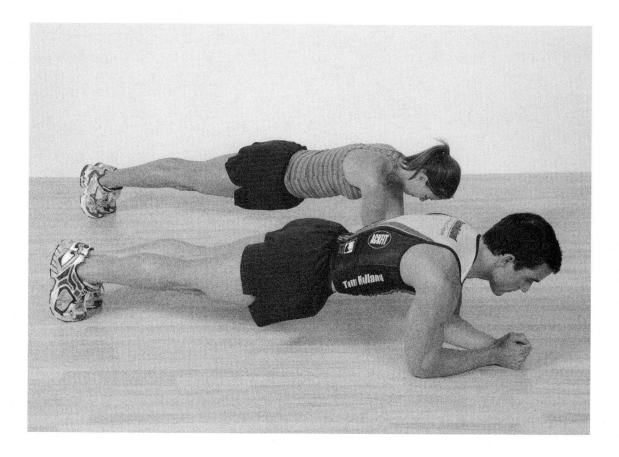

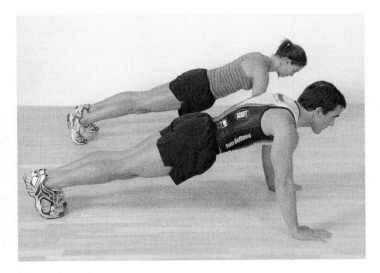

BUILD PHASE

Push-ups
Muscle focus: Chest
Sets: 2
Reps: To failure

Regular push-ups. Beginners may start on knees and progress to full push-ups. Lower down slowly until your chest is a few inches off of the floor, then return to starting position.

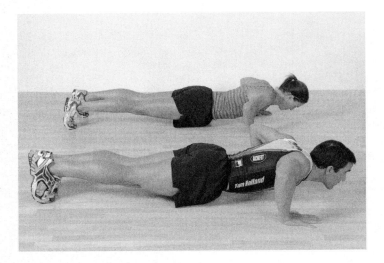

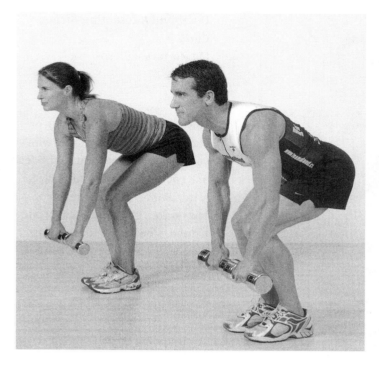

Dumbbell Bent-Over Rows— Bent Arms
Muscle focus: Back
Sets: 2
Reps: 12

Bend at the waist until your upper body is parallel to the floor with your knees bent. Hold the dumbbells under your chest with arms extended and palms facing behind you. Keeping your back flat, slowly raise the weights until your elbows are just above your shoulders and your arms are bent to 90 degrees, hold for one second, then lower back to starting position.

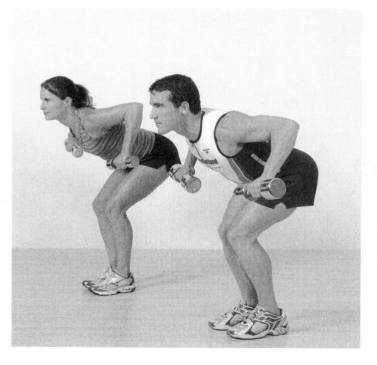

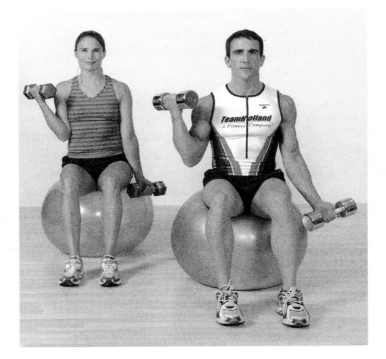

Dumbbell Alternating Biceps Curls

Muscle focus: Biceps
Sets: 2
Reps: 12 each arm

This may be done while sitting or standing. Hold the dumbbell with your elbows tucked in to your sides and your palms facing naturally forward. Slowly raise one weight up toward your shoulder, hold for one second, slowly lower back down, then repeat with the other arm. This equals one repetition.

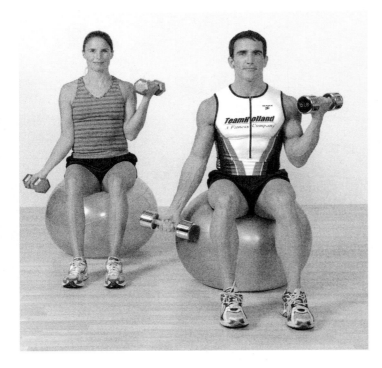

Dumbbell Front and Side Raises
Muscle focus: Shoulders
Sets: 2
Reps: 12

Stand in a split stance with one leg in front of the other and your knees slightly bent. Holding the dumbbells at tops of thighs, with your elbows slightly bent, slowly raise them in front of you to your shoulder height, hold for one second, then slowly lower. Next, slowly raise the weights out to your sides with elbows slightly bent, up to shoulder height, hold for one second, then lower back to starting position. This is one repetition.

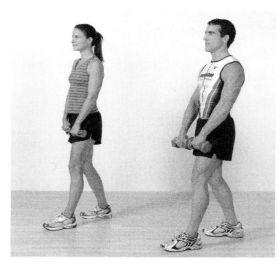 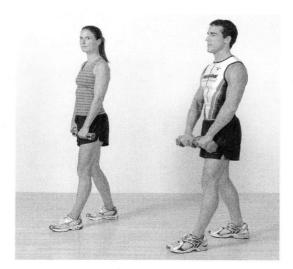

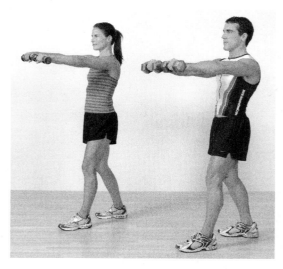 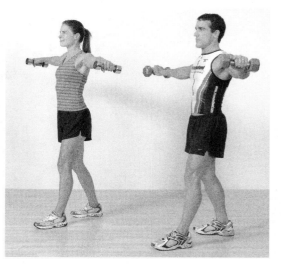

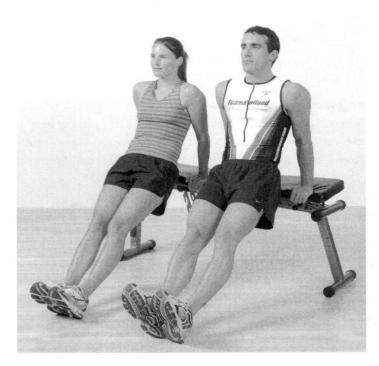

Triceps Bench Dips

Muscle focus: Triceps
Sets: 2
Reps: 12

Position yourself on the side of a bench or chair with your back to it, holding yourself up with your hands on the edge. With knees bent, slowly bend your elbows and lower your body down to the floor several inches, hold for one second, then push yourself back up until your arms are fully extended once again.

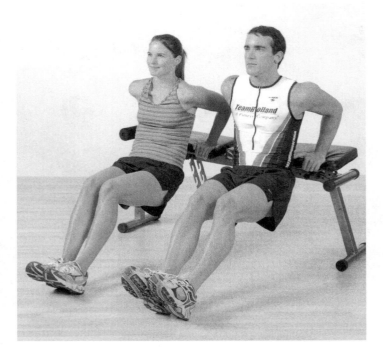

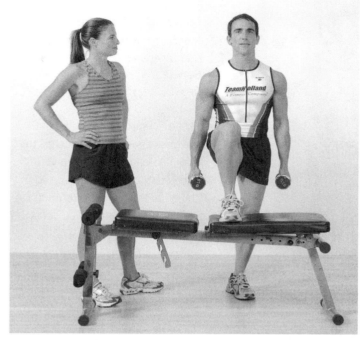

Bench Step Ups
(dumbbells optional)

Muscle focus: Glutes, hamstrings, quadriceps

Sets: 2

Reps: 12

Place your right foot on a bench no higher than knee height. Step up and tap your left foot on the bench while fully extending your right leg, step back down with the left leg, then immediately repeat.

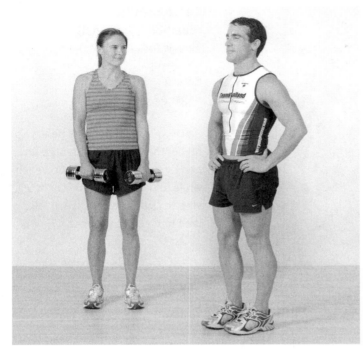

Front Lunges
(dumbbells optional)

Muscle focus: Glutes, hamstrings, quadriceps
Sets: 2
Reps: 12 each leg

Stride forward with one leg until the back knee almost touches the floor, making sure to keep your knees behind your toes and your chest up. Push off and return to the starting position.

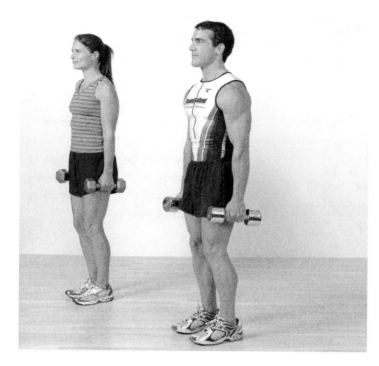

Back Lunges
(dumbbells optional)

Muscle focus: Glutes, hamstrings, quadriceps

Sets: 2
Reps: 12

Stride backward with one leg until the back knee almost touches the floor, making sure to keep your knees behind your toes and your chest up. Push off and return to the starting position.

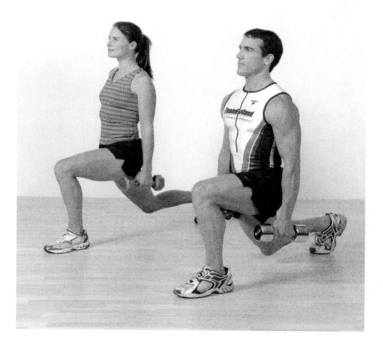

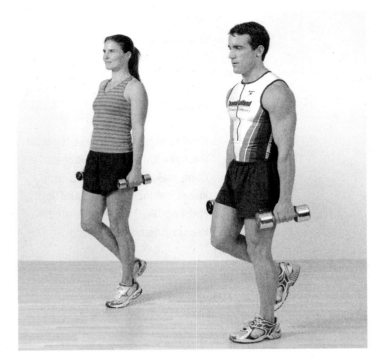

Single Leg Calf Raises
(dumbbell optional)
Muscle focus: Calves
Sets: 2
Reps: 12 each leg

Stand on one foot, the other leg raised slightly in the air, holding on to something for support. Raise your body up in the air by standing on your toes, then lower back down to starting position.

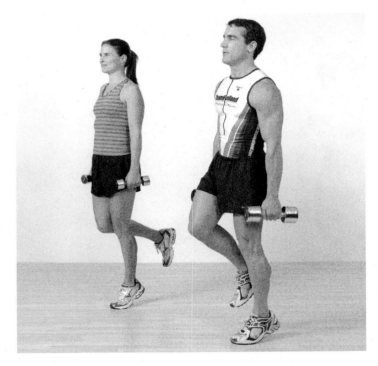

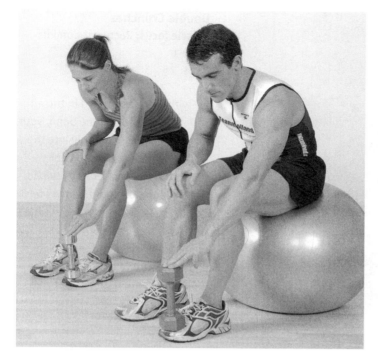

Single Leg Dumbbell Toe Raises

Muscle focus: Shins
Sets: 2
Reps: 12 each leg

Sit on a chair or bench with one hand holding a dumbbell balanced on your toes. Lift the dumbbell up in the air by curling your toes toward your shin, then lower back to starting position.

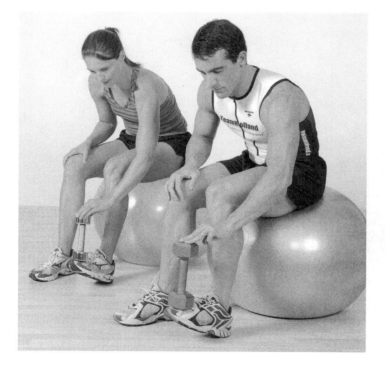

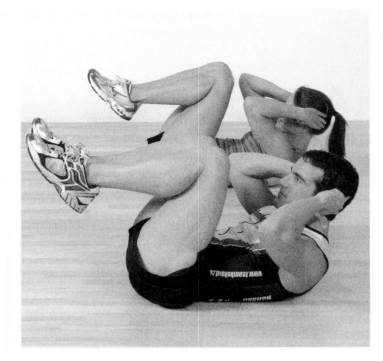

Double Crunches

Muscle focus: Rectus abdominis
Sets: 1
Reps: 25

Lie with your feet raised in the air with 90 degrees of knee bend, your lower back pressed firmly into the floor, your hands behind your head, and your upper body raised. Making sure to keep the lower back down, reach away from your body with your feet until your legs are almost fully extended, and lower your upper body to the floor, hold for one second, then return to starting position.

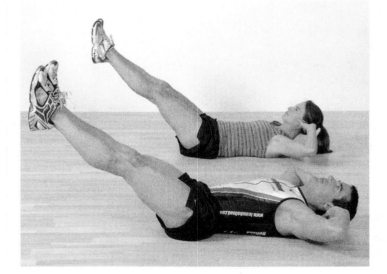

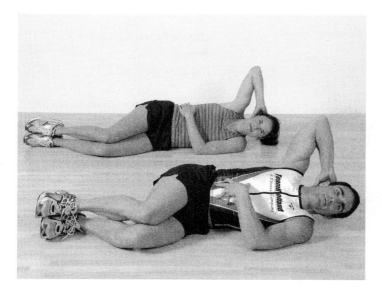

Knee Down Oblique Twists

Muscle focus: Obliques
Sets: 1
Reps: 25 each side

Lie on your side with both knees bent and on the floor to your left. With your right hand behind your head, bring your right elbow toward your right hip and hold for one second, then lower back down a few inches and repeat.

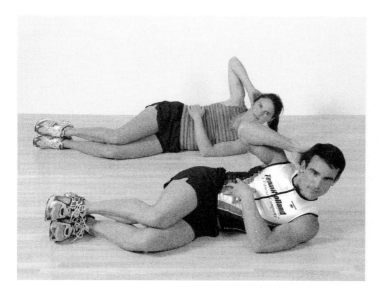

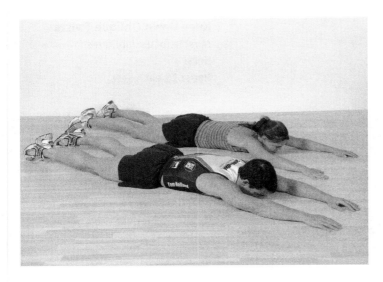

Swim

Muscle focus: Spinal erectors
Sets: 1
Reps: 12 each side

Lie on your stomach with your arms straight above your head. Simultaneously lift your left hand and your right leg up off the floor, squeezing the muscles of your lower back; hold for one second, then slowly lower back down and repeat with the other arm and leg. This equals one repetition.

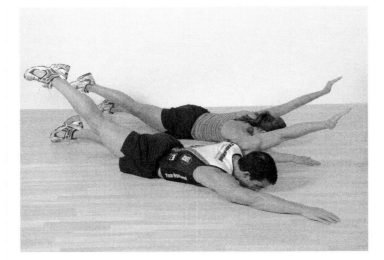

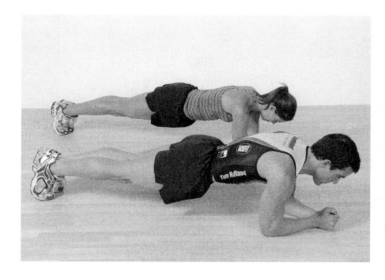

Raised Leg Plank

Muscle focus: Abdominals and lower back
Sets: 1
Reps: 1 minute

Assume a push-up position but support your upper body with your forearms and your palms pressed together. Keep your body perfectly straight and your abdominals tight, yet breathe normally. Raise one leg and hold for a three count, then switch legs. Continue to alternate for one minute.

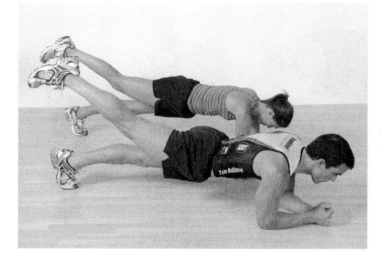

Plank

Muscle focus: Abdominals and lower back
Sets: 1
Reps: 1 minute

Assume a push-up position but support your upper body with your forearms and your palms pressed together. Keep your body perfectly straight and your abdominals tight, yet breathe normally. Hold this position for one minute.

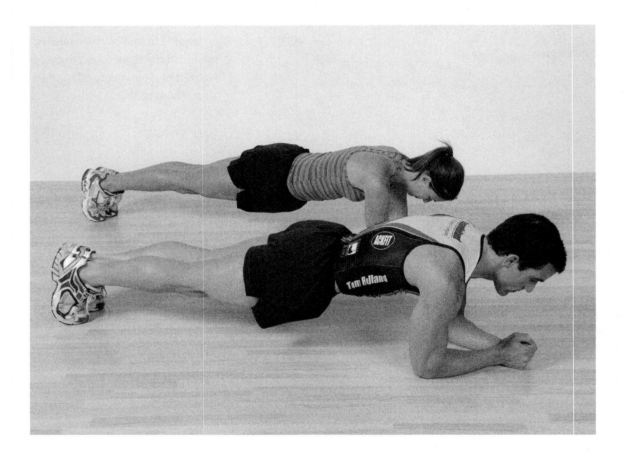

PEAK PHASE

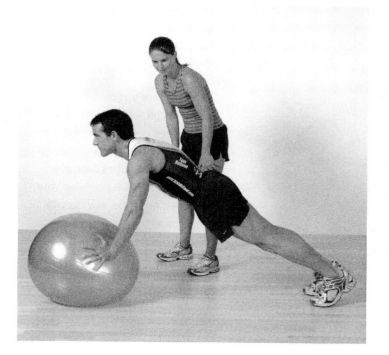

Stability Ball Push-ups
Muscle focus: Chest, shoulders, triceps, and core
Sets: 3
Reps: To failure

Place a stability ball against a wall for support and assume a push-up position with your hands on the ball. Slowly lower yourself down until your chest is a few inches from the ball, then push back up.

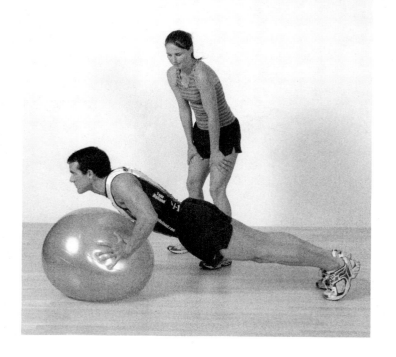

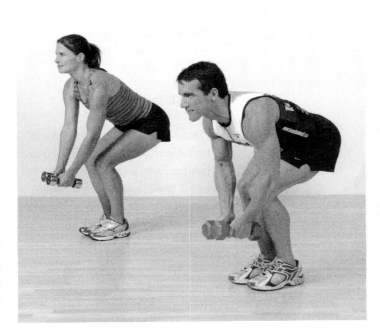

Dumbbell Bent-Over Flys
Muscle focus: Back
Sets: 2
Reps: 12

Bend at the waist until your upper body is parallel to the floor, with your knees bent. Hold the dumbbells under your chest with arms extended and palms facing together. Making sure to keep your back flat, raise the weights with a slight bend in your elbows out to the side until they are in line with your shoulders, hold for one second, then lower.

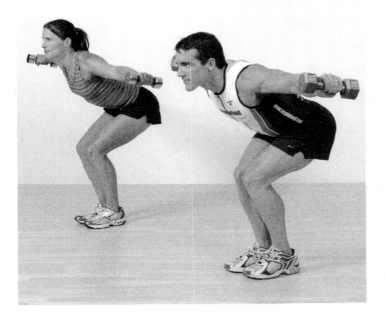

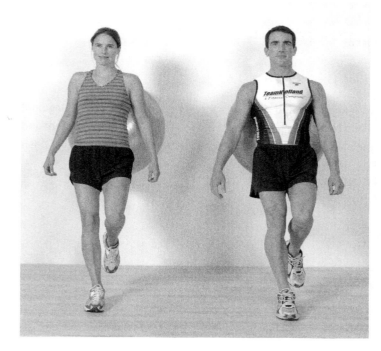

Single Leg Stability Ball Squats (dumbbells optional)

Muscle focus: Glutes, hamstrings, quadriceps
Sets: 2
Reps: 15

Stand on one leg while pressing a stability ball into a wall with your back. Keeping your chest up and knees behind your toes, lower your body down to just above 90 degrees of knee bend, hold for one second, then return to starting position.

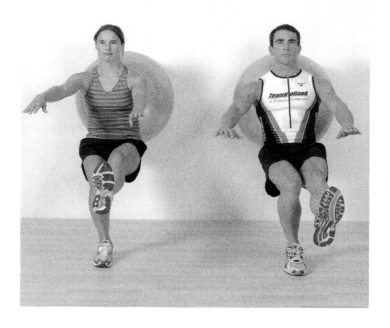

Front and Back Lunges Combo
(dumbbells optional)

Muscle focus: Glutes, hamstrings, quadriceps
Sets: 2
Reps: 15 each leg

Making sure to keep your chest up and your knees behind your toes, step forward with your right leg until the back knee almost touches the floor, return to starting position without touching the foot to the floor and then immediately stride backward until the back knee almost touches the floor, return to the starting position and repeat.

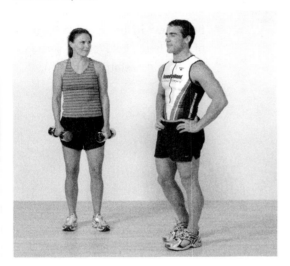
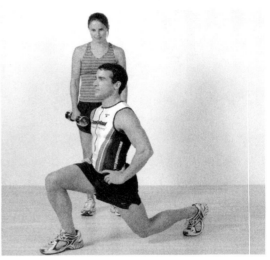

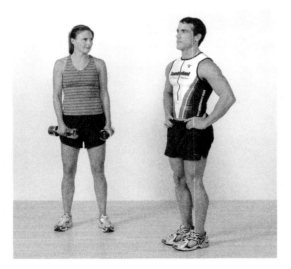
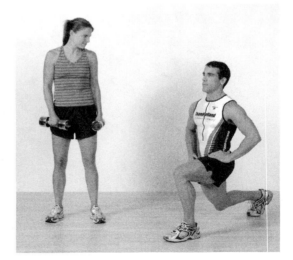

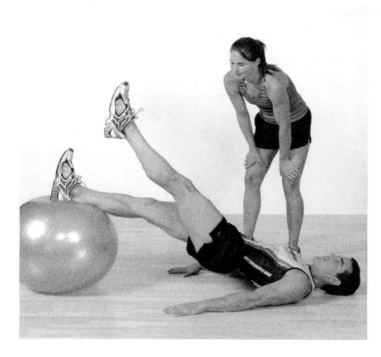

Single Leg Stability Ball Hamstring Curls

Muscle focus: Hamstrings, core
Sets: 2
Reps: 15 each leg

Lie with your back on the floor with your hips raised and one heel on the stability ball. Pull the ball with this leg to your butt, then return to starting position. Do not allow your hips to touch the floor throughout the exercise.

Stability Ball Wall Sit (dumbbells optional)

Muscle focus: Glutes, hamstrings, quadriceps
Sets: 2
Reps: 1 minute

Stand while pressing a stability ball into a wall with your back. Your feet should be a little wider than shoulder width apart, with your toes pointing forward. Keeping your chest up and knees behind your toes, lower your body down to just above 90 degrees of knee bend and hold for one minute.

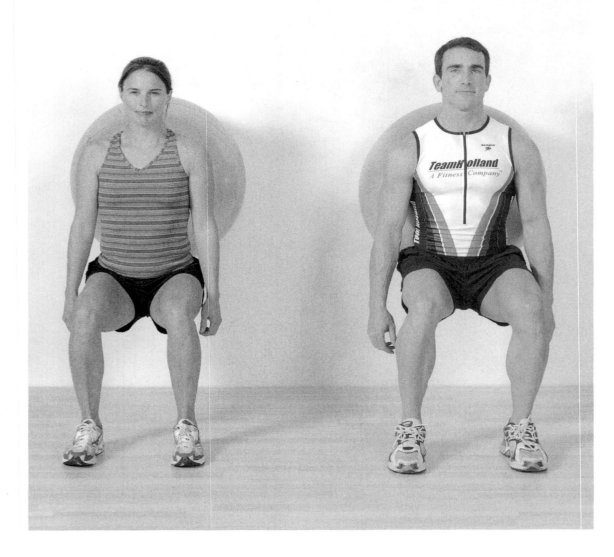

Stability Ball Reverse Crunches

Muscle focus: Core
Sets: 2
Reps: 15

Assume a push-up position with your feet on a stability ball. Pull the ball toward you while keeping your hips high in the air, then return to start position.

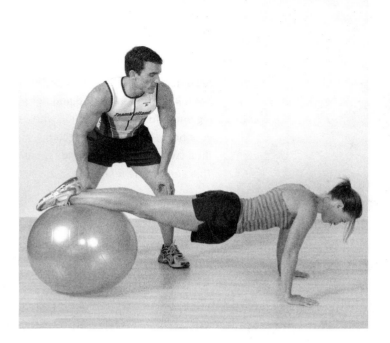

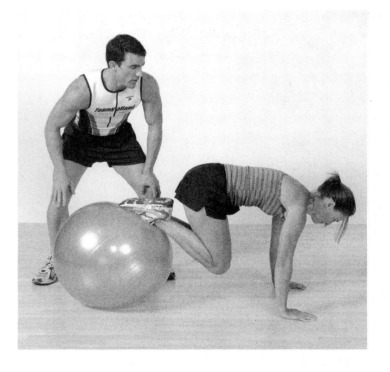

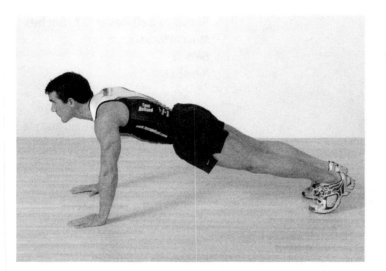

Two-Point Bridge
Muscle focus: Core
Sets: 1
Reps: 5

Assume a push-up position and hold. Raise your left hand and right leg out to form a straight line with your body, hold for a three count, then switch arm and leg and repeat. This equals one repetition.

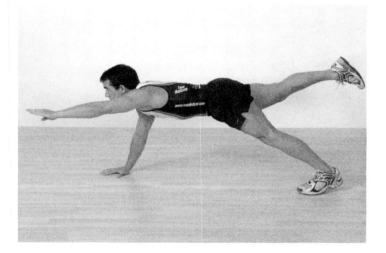

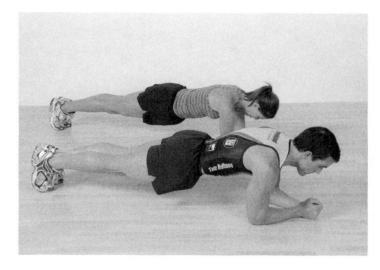

Plank
Muscle focus: Core
Sets: 1
Reps: 2 minutes

Assume a push-up position but support your upper body with your forearms and your palms pressed together. Keep your body perfectly straight and your abdominals tight, yet breathe normally. Hold this position for two minutes.

THE CORE

Working the "core" has become increasingly popular over the years, and for good reason. These muscles that comprise the anterior and posterior abdominal area, or front and back of your middle, are really important to both sports performance and daily functional strength. Different fitness professionals may define the core with greater or fewer muscles, but for our purposes they include: the rectus abdominis, the obliques, the transverse abdominis, and the spinal erectors. A weak core means potential injury and decreased performance. Core strength is extremely important in triathlon, helping you to maintain optimal body position during the swim, to hold the aero position for long periods of time on the bike, and to maintain proper form during the run, as well as for allowing the optimal transfer of power throughout your entire body.

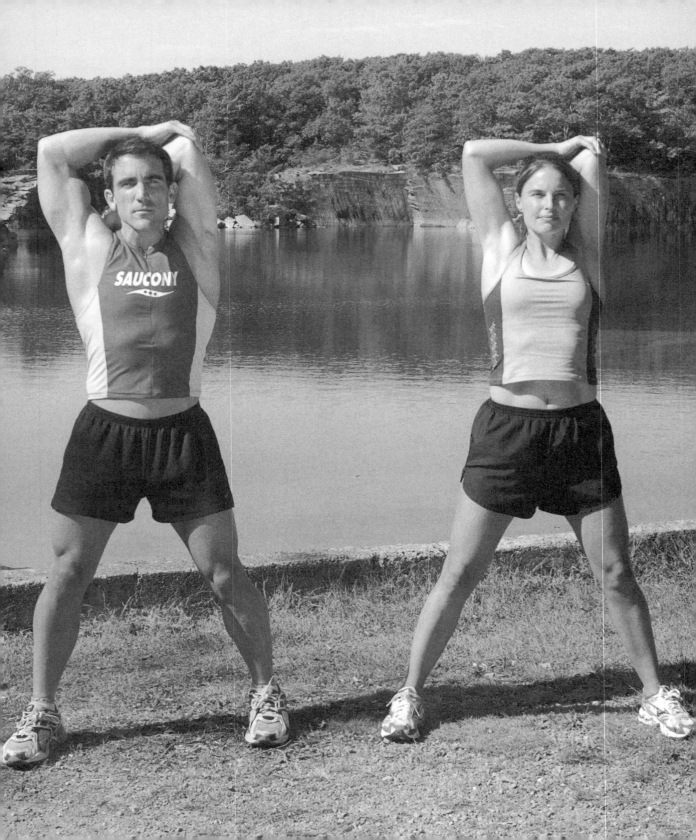

CHAPTER 5
Stretching and Flexibility Program

It still amazes me how many articles are out there that state that stretching either does not help prevent injury and/or will not improve sport performance. I disagree, as do countless professional athletes.

GUIDELINES FOR STRETCHING

There is also conflicting information about when and how much to stretch. Well, the most current research in favor of stretching suggests the following three steps:

1. Begin with roughly a three- to five-minute "dynamic warm-up" before stretching. For example, this means that prior to a run session, you should ideally run easy for three to five minutes before you begin to stretch. The reason for this is that you want to warm up your muscles first before stretching. The goal is to increase the blood flow gradually to the muscles you will be using, through a low-intensity warm-up. You can, in fact, pull a muscle during your stretch session if you try to force a cold muscle too far too soon.

2. After this dynamic warm-up, you should stop and stretch the major muscles that you will be using, holding these stretches for roughly ten to fifteen seconds. So, before your run workout, you will run easy for a few minutes, then stop and stretch such muscles as your quadriceps (front of your thighs), hamstrings (back of your thighs), calves, glutes, and any muscles including those of the upper body that may be tight. This whole stretch should take but a few minutes, tops.

3. Then, after your run session, you will perform the same stretches once again, but this time, you will hold each stretch for thirty to sixty seconds. Your muscles should now be really warmed up, and you will have a greater range of motion than you had just a short time ago before you began your workout.

The dynamic warm-up can be any gradual exercise that gets the blood flowing to the muscles you are about to use. Running in place, jumping jacks, whatever; as long as it slowly increases your heart rate. Obviously, the best warm-up would consist of movements that are close to the movements that you are about to perform.

You know those men and women you may have made fun of, who bounce, hop, and skip around before their running or triathlon races? The ones who do those short sprints just prior to the gun going off? Remember how you thought, "How stupid, they are wasting valuable energy?" Now you know it's their dynamic warm-up, not just some wacky prerace ritual. And most of those people are the first ones over the finish line, as well.

STRETCHES

Stretching is one of those things that doesn't take a long time to do, yet I believe pays incredible dividends to performance, injury prevention, and sports longevity. Like everything else, the key is consistency, not quantity.

1. Standing Quadriceps Stretch

Stand upright and hold the toes of one foot as you gently pull your heel toward your butt. Keep both knees side by side; do not pull the leg back behind you or lean forward. You can bend your supporting leg slightly. You should feel a gentle stretch in the front of your raised thigh. Do this with both legs.

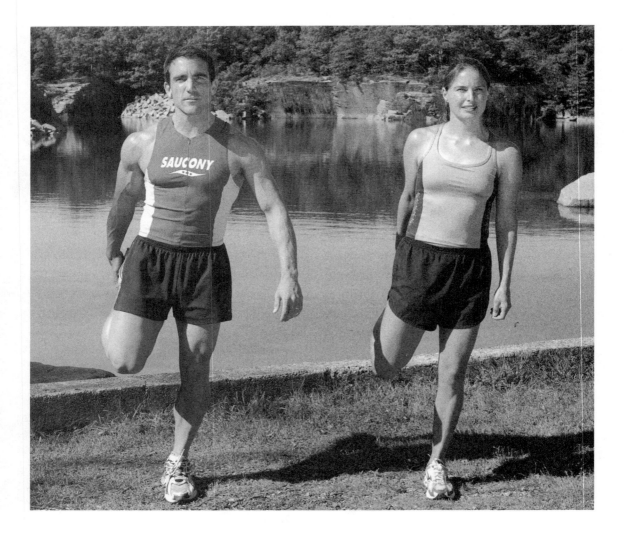

2. Standing Hamstring Stretch

Stand with legs spread apart and your hands resting on one thigh. Gradually shift your weight onto the leg you are holding and press down on that same foot. You should feel a gentle stretch in the back of your thigh. Do this with both legs.

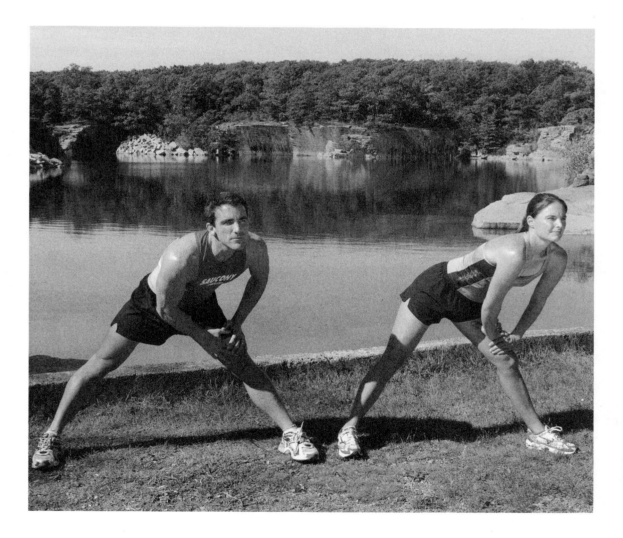

3. Standing Calf Stretch

Stand in a split stance with your hands on your front thigh; keep your back leg straight. Gently press the heel of your back leg down into the ground while bending your front knee slowly forward. You should feel a gentle stretch in the back of your lower leg. Do this with both legs.

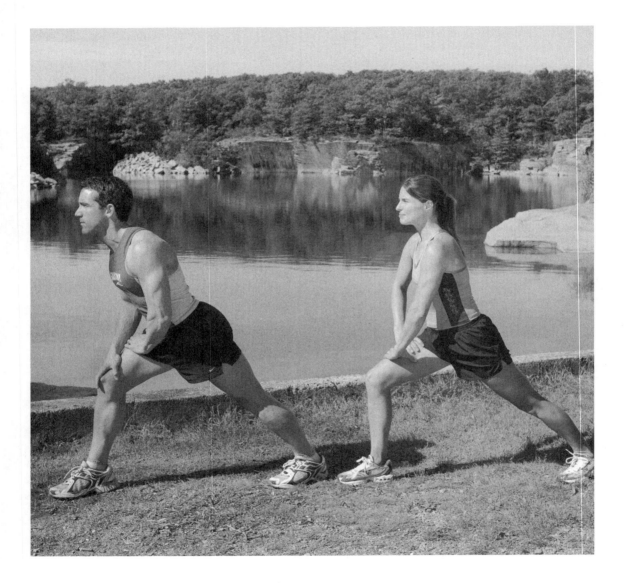

4. Standing Glute Stretch

Holding on to an object such as a chair or bench for support, or balancing with your hands on your leg, cross one ankle above your knee and slowly sit back as if you were lowering yourself down into a seated position. Stop when you feel a gentle stretch in the glute (butt) of the leg that is raised and hold. Do this with both legs.

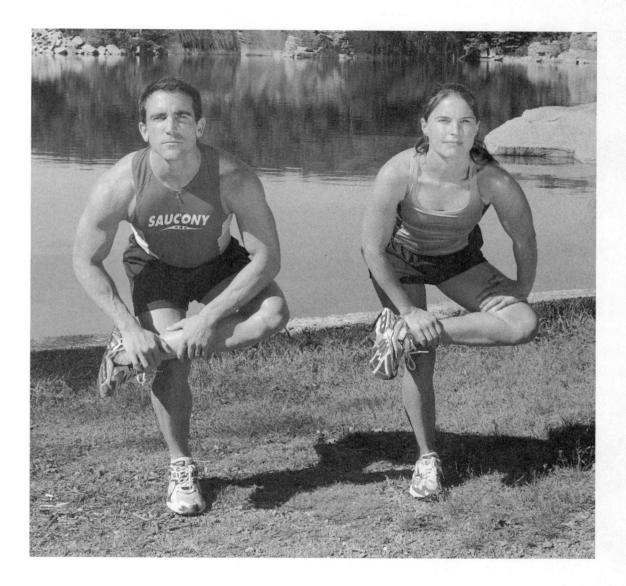

5. Standing Adductor Stretch

Stand with feet wider than shoulder width apart and toes open. Place your hands on the thigh of one leg and bend that knee out to the side as you straighten the opposite leg. Press down on the foot of the leg that is straight as you bend, stopping movement and holding when you feel a gentle stretch on the inside of the thigh of the straightened leg. Do this to both sides.

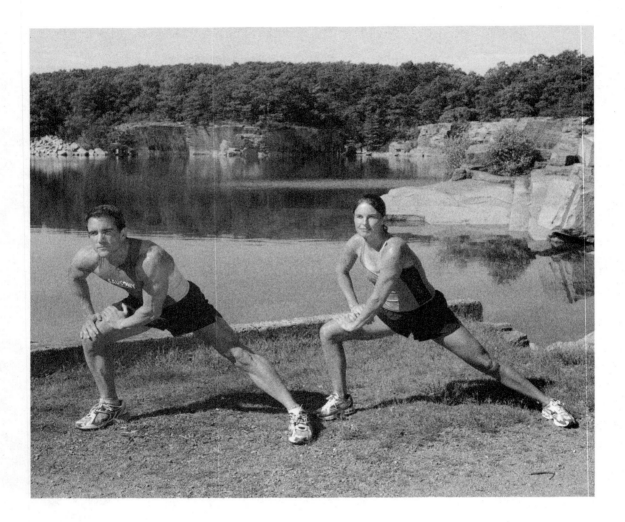

6. Standing Upper Body Stretch (Shoulders, triceps, back)

Bend one arm behind your head and place the palm of that hand against your upper back. Grasp the elbow with your free hand and slowly pull it away from the shoulder until you feel a gentle stretch, then hold. Do this with both arms.

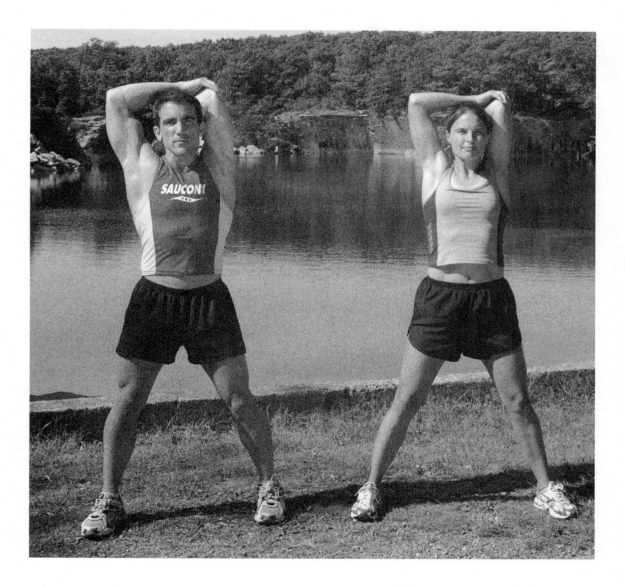

7. Standing Neck Stretch

Placing one hand on the side of your head, gradually drop your ear toward your shoulder while pulling down very gently on your head until you feel the stretch, and hold. Do this to both sides.

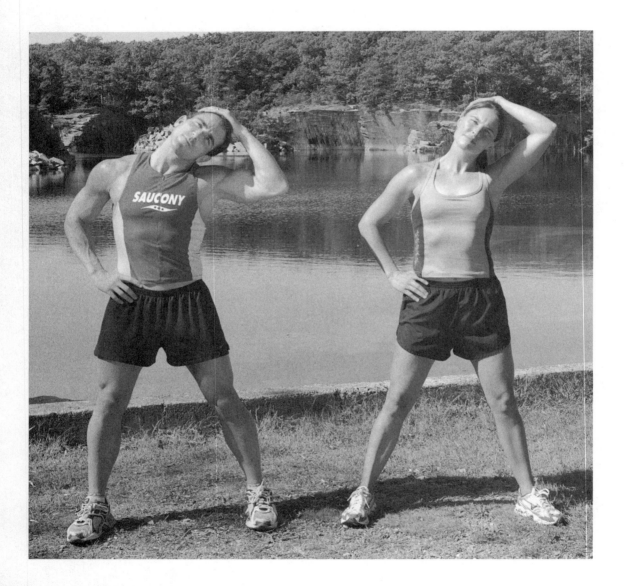

8. Standing Hamstring Stretch #2

Stand in a split stance with one leg out straight, heel on the ground and your hands resting on this thigh. Gradually lean forward and press down on this heel until you feel a gentle stretch behind the thigh of the leg you are holding. Do this with both legs.

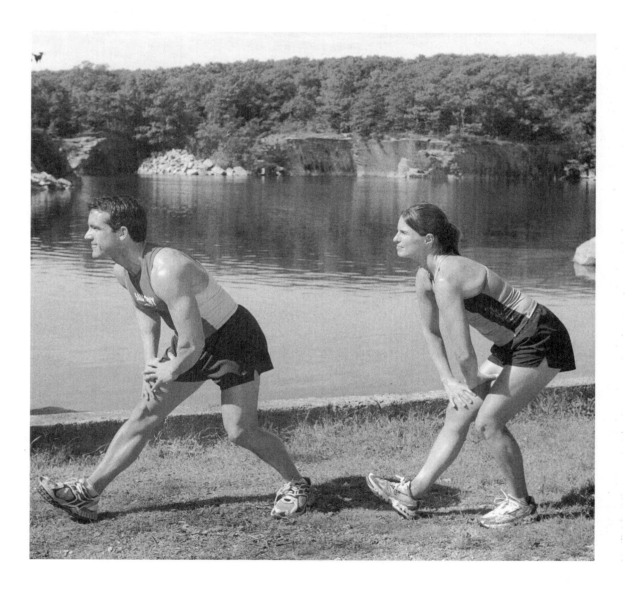

9. Standing Groin Stretch

Stand with feet spread wide apart. Gradually spread your legs farther and farther apart while lowering your upper body toward the floor. Placing your hands on the floor for support, spread your legs until you feel a gentle stretch on the inside of both thighs, and hold. Make sure your footing is secure and not too slippery.

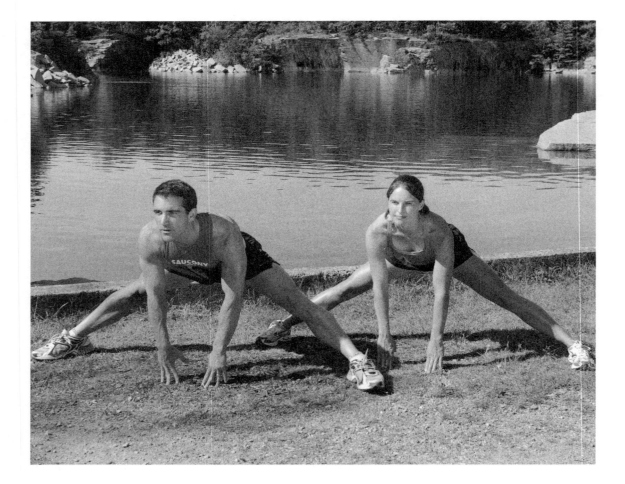

10. Standing Lower Back Stretch

Stand with legs just wider than shoulder width apart and knees slightly bent. Place your hands on your right hip and slowly rotate your upper body to the right and hold. You should feel a gentle stretch in your lower back. Do this on both sides.

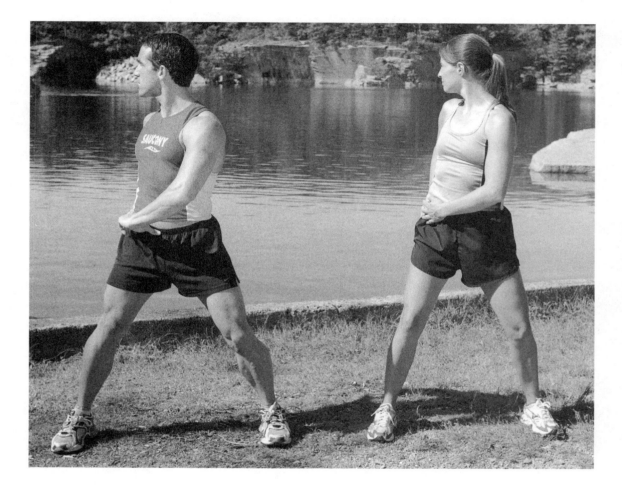

If you do all of these stretches and hold them each for 30 seconds, the entire routine should take you only nine minutes to complete. There are two hamstring stretches to choose from, as I like to do these both when I stretch, but you can choose one each session and alternate them. So you really have only around eight minutes of stretching to do. Our hamstrings can become really tight from triathlon training, and this tightness can lead to a bunch of problems, so pay particular attention to this muscle group!

Yes, there are many more stretches that can be performed and many variations on how you can stretch each individual muscle group. My goal is not to give you everything, but to give you just enough of the really effective stuff so that you do it. Remember: It's quality, not quantity—and consistency!

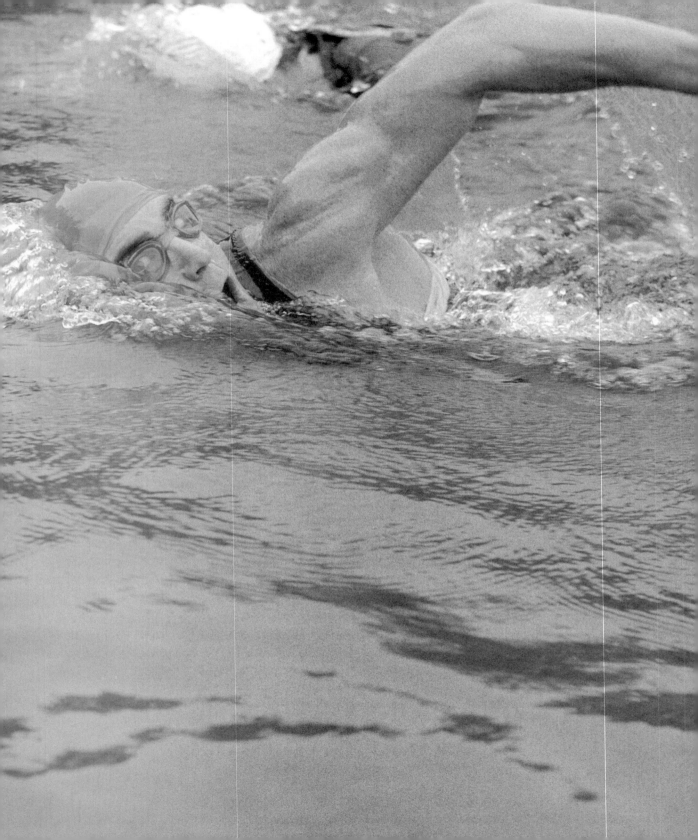

CHAPTER 6
Swim Training

Ask most people who have never participated in a triathlon why they have not and they inevitably reply, "I could do the bike and the run; it's the swim that scares the heck out of me." Someone put it perfectly when they remarked that swimming is not a sport, it is merely a means to keep from drowning. The swim leg of triathlon does frighten many people, and to be honest, this fear is quite understandable. If you get tired or panic during the bike or the run, you slow down, you stop. This is not as easy to do during the swim portion of a triathlon. Also, it is almost impossible to replicate the race-day conditions of the swim during your training. Unless you have several hundred friends who are willing to swim next to you in the open water during your swim sessions, you will not be able to truly simulate the race-day conditions you will find in most triathlons. More likely you will do the majority of your swim training in the safe confines of a pool, with lane lines on either side of you, where you can stand if you need to, get out whenever you wish, and see the bottom (hopefully!), and where the odds of a shark or other creature swimming next to you are extremely low. I will discuss swim strategies more in the later section on racing, especially the sport psychology end of it, but know that the more confident you are in your swimming, the less nervous you will be during the swim.

I consider swimming to be analogous to golf in that it's about technique, technique, technique. It doesn't matter how fit you are, the more unfit person with a superior swim stroke will fly by you in a race. You cannot "muscle" your way through to a fast swim. The main factor slowing you down is water resistance, and lessening the effects of this resistance comes down to technique, namely such concepts as body position, body rotation, the arm pull, and the kick.

When I started out in triathlon, I read numerous books and articles on swimming and came to the realization that it is extremely difficult to learn how to swim by reading about it. The descriptions of the specific drills and pointers on correct technique are very hard to pull off of the page and translate into real-world mechanics. For this reason, I suggest you do the following to improve your swim technique.

1. *Hire a coach.* Invest in several sessions with a qualified swim coach. Try to find one who is familiar with swimming as it applies to triathlon; the money spent will be well worth it. Ideally, he or she will observe you as you swim in a pool and begin to make the necessary modifications to your stroke. Also have the coach demonstrate several drills for you to incorporate into your swim sessions. After a few initial sessions with a coach, train for a month or

so on your own and then meet with the coach again to monitor your progress, further refine your stroke, and demonstrate new drills to add to your repertoire. Don't try to take on too much too soon; like golf, swimming generally requires one or two small changes to be mastered before you can move on to the next modification in technique. We can focus on only a limited number of tasks at a time, and attempting to change too many things at once is extremely difficult.

2. *Purchase several instructional swim videos.* There are numerous quality swim videos that you can use to drastically improve your stroke. Again, many people are visual learners, and these videos will allow you to see the correct form as it is described. The mind is a powerful tool, and by watching the correct form repeated over and over, you will engrave the patterns in your mind. This is much more advantageous than swimming hard repeats in the pool with crummy form. Remember that practicing swimming poorly will only make you a better crummy swimmer. Total Immersion is one of the leaders in quality instructional swim videos, and I recommend them highly: www.TotalImmersion.net.

3. *Join a master's swim team.* Many local YMCAs, YWCAs, and other swim facilities have master's swim teams that you should consider joining if you truly want to improve your swim technique. Many are coached by highly qualified swimmers who take the group through structured workouts several times a week. Adding at least one weekly master's swim team practice into your training will pay dividends in your swim performance. Here you will experience some of the tension that you will encounter during a race as you will be swimming several people in a lane and you will have the pressure of trying to keep up with the pace of those around you.

For those of you who will be following the Finish programs, you will simply swim by time. It's that simple. Your goal is to get through that swim intact and get onto your bike.

If you can swim without stopping for the longest of your 12-Week Triathlete program's swim workout, then you will physically be able to finish the swim leg of your triathlon.

You can choose to structure this swim workout however you choose; the goal is for you to build up your endurance as well as confidence so that you can complete the swim leg of your triathlon.

As you strive to improve your swim stroke and lower your swim times, you may want to utilize specific training aids to further enhance your technique. The following are commonly used during portions of swim sessions to improve specific elements of the swim stroke:

TRAINING GEAR

1. *Fins:* These help improve ankle flexibility, increase your kick strength, and help you to "ride high" in the water, especially during drills.

2. *Paddles:* These help to develop correct hand entry and optimize extension and tracking during the catch and pull phases of the freestyle swim stroke.

3. *Pull buoy:* Helps to maintain proper body positioning.
4. *Kickboard:* You remember these from when we were kids. You use these to help improve and strengthen your kick.

Many pools have kickboards and pull buoys that you can borrow during your swim workouts. You will most likely have to buy your own fins and paddles if you choose to use them.

How many laps do I have to swim to make a mile in the pool?

Pools are usually twenty-five meters or twenty-five yards long (yards and meters are used interchangeably for the most part when designing swim workouts), with the bigger pools being twice the distance or fifty meters long. One length of the pool is from one end to the other; one lap is down and back. In a twenty-five-meter-long pool, one mile would be swimming thirty-five laps or seventy lengths of the pool.

Do I have to swim freestyle in the triathlon? If I need to take a break, can I switch to breaststroke or backstroke or is that against the rules?

You can swim whatever stroke you want, whenever you want. People swim freestyle because that is what most people can swim the fastest and the easiest, but there is no rule that says you must swim a certain stroke. If you can swim the butterfly faster than you can swim the freestyle, then you go right ahead.

STRUCTURED WORKOUTS

A simple way to structure your swim workouts is as follows:

1. *Warm-up:* Easy swim. Some people do their drills during their warm-up; others simply swim easy to get the blood flowing and loosen up the muscles.
2. *Drills:* Examples would be fingertip-drag drills, fists, catch-up, kicking with the kickboard, swimming with the pull buoy, swimming with the paddles, bilateral

SWIM DISTANCE CHART

DISTANCE (miles)	DISTANCE (yards)	LAPS (25-yard pool)*
.25	440	9
.5	880	18
.95	1,672	34
1	1,760	35
1.2	2,112	43
2	3,520	71
2.4	4,224	85

* laps rounded up

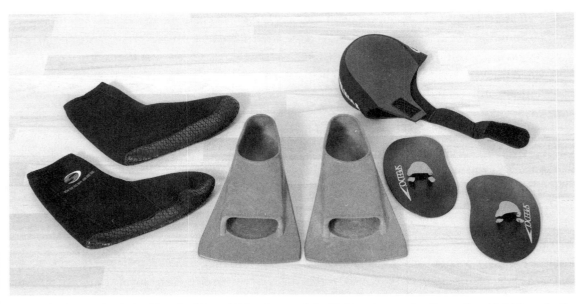

Pictured left to right: Swim "booties" for additional warmth in frigid waters; swim fins; a "squid lid," again, for additional warmth in frigid waters; and swim paddles

breathing (breathing to both sides), one-armed drills, and many more. Again, in my opinion, the only real way to learn these drills is to see them being performed correctly by a private coach, in a master's swim session, or by watching a swim video like those made by Total Immersion. If you truly want to improve your swimming, then you should spend a large chunk of your swim session practicing these drills to improve your form. Remember, swimming for an hour poorly will only reinforce swimming poorly.

3. *Intervals:* During interval workouts, you will break up your swim into different distances, strokes, intensities, and the time you spend resting in between "sets." "Sets" might look like the following swim workout prescribed to me by my coach years ago:

W/UP 400, 5 × (300-200-100
ON 10 SR), COOLDOWN

During this workout, you would warm up for 400 yards, then swim 200 yards, rest for 10 seconds, and repeat this 5 times. Then you would swim 200 yards, rest for 10 seconds, and repeat this 5 times. Then you would swim 100 yards, rest for 10 seconds, and repeat this 5 times, then cool down for a few hundred yards. This is a fairly simple and straightforward workout.

If you do the math, you will realize that this is about 4,000 yards of swimming, or almost 2¼ miles. That's a great deal of swimming for most people! Unless you are really looking to improve your swimming and/or your race is a long-distance triathlon, you do not have to swim this much during your swim workouts. This workout was designed for higher performance at the Ironman distance.

I could prescribe swim workouts of many thousands of yards that are highly complex and contain varying intensities, but these workouts are beneficial to a select few, in my experience, and you can and will benefit by doing much less.

4. *Cool-Down:* Easy swim.

So, in say a 30-minute swim session, you may warm up for 5 minutes, do 5 to 10 minutes of drills, spend 15 to 25 minutes doing interval work, and then have 5 to 10 minutes of cooling down.

The pool where I swim has workouts on the board that we can follow, but I am confused— what does "4 × 200 free on 3:30, 3:25, 3:20, 3:15" mean?

Most pools have a large clock or two that are "pace clocks." They time in 60-second intervals, and you use these to time your sets. So, for the above-mentioned workout, you would time yourself as you swim the first 200 yards. If you finish in 3 minutes flat, then you have 15 seconds to rest since you are allowed a total time of 3:30. For the second 200, if you finish in 3:20, then you would have only 5 seconds to rest.

SAMPLE SWIM SETS

For those of you who will be following the Performance training plans, you may select from the following swim workouts depending on your overall swim time and the time you have chosen to devote to technique drills. Mix them up and add the occasional straight long swim in as well. If you wish to swim a main set longer than 2,000 yards, you can simply add in additional intervals. These are but a few ways to structure your swim workouts.

MAIN SET: 500 YARDS

1. 10 × 50 @ 15 sec rest
2. 3 × 100 @ 20 sec rest/4 × 50 @ 15 sec rest
3. 2 × 200 @ 20 sec rest/2 × 50 @ 10 sec rest
4. 200/2 × 100 @ 15 sec rest/
   50/2 × 25 @ 10 sec rest
5. 50/100/200/100/50 @ 15 sec rest

MAIN SET: 1,000 YARDS

1. 5 × 200 @ 20 sec rest
2. 500 @ 30 sec rest/5 × 100 @ 15 sec rest
3. 100/200/400/200/100 @ 20 sec rest
4. 2 × 500 @ 30 sec rest
5. 3 × 300 @ 25 sec rest/4 × 25
   @ 5 sec rest

MAIN SET: 2,000 YARDS

1. 10 × 100 @ 15 sec rest/
   2 × 500 @ 30 sec rest
2. 100/200/300/2 × 400/300/200/100
   @ 20 sec rest
3. 4 × 500 @ 25 sec rest
4. 10 × 100 @ 10 sec rest/4 × 200
   @ 25 sec rest/8 × 25 @ 10 sec rest
5. 10 × 50 @ 15 sec rest/2 × 500
   @ 30 sec rest/5 × 100 @ 10 sec rest

Try to make each interval a little stronger than the one before, and learn to pace yourself.

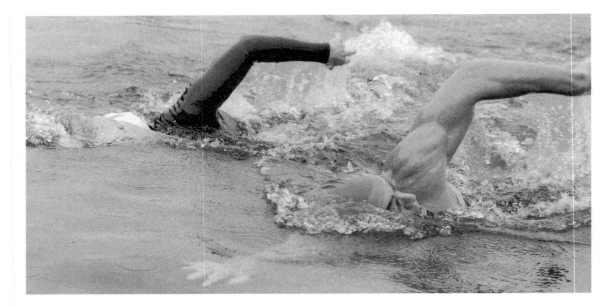

If you push too hard and fatigue early, your stroke will suffer in the later intervals.

You may also choose to alter the workouts by designating certain intervals as kick sets, sets with the pull buoy, and so forth. As you get closer to your race, your intervals should ideally decrease in length and increase in intensity.

OPEN WATER SWIMMING

As I stated at the beginning of the chapter, this is the aspect of triathlon that strikes the most fear into people, and this fear is commonly cited as the reason why someone has not participated in one. This makes complete sense. Open water swimming can be very stressful, especially in the larger races where it starts with a mass swim start rather than a wave start.

Mass swim start: All athletes start the race together. This can be very hectic, as swimmers generally fight for position in the water—there is contact between swimmers.

Wave swim start: Swimmers start in "waves," groups that are often determined by age groups and separated by starts of under a minute to several minutes. The pros may go first, then the 18- to 24-year-olds, then 25- to 29, and so on. Your finishing time is adjusted at the end according to your specific wave start.

Open water swimming is a unique aspect of triathlon in the sense that the majority of athletes will not be training in these conditions much, if at all. Think about it: the conditions of your training for the bike and the run will most likely be quite similar come race day. This is rarely the case when it comes to the swim. Most people will train for the swim by performing lap workouts in the pool, and unless your triathlon swim is in the pool (yes, some are!), your race-day conditions in the open water will be markedly different. These conditions may include, but are not limited to, the following: You may be swimming with a large group of people,

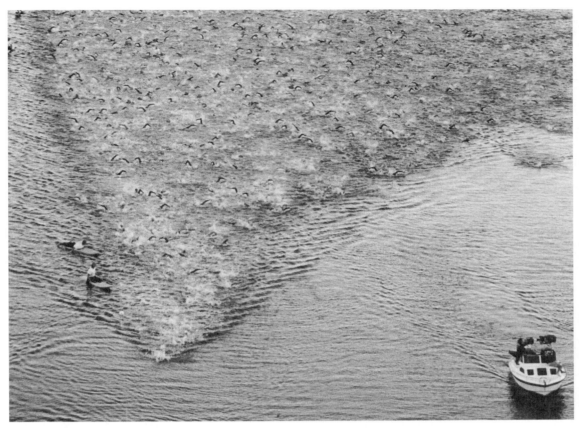

2002 Ironman Australia Mass Swim Start

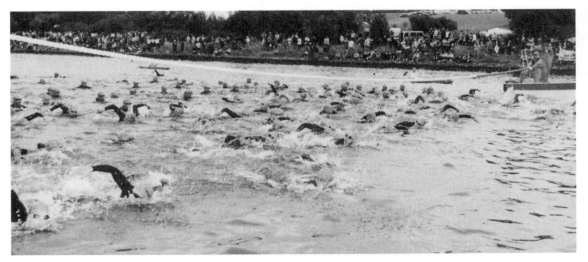

1999 Ironman Germany Wave Swim Start

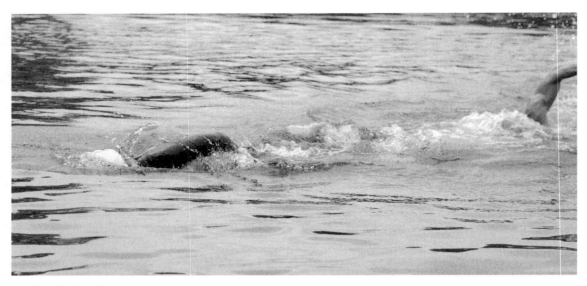

Drafting during the swim.

and body contact is common; you may be in a wetsuit; you might not be able to see the bottom; you don't have a wall to grab on to or push off of; waves may be an issue; marine life, big and small, real or imagined, may be an issue; and you will have to "sight" to see where you are going.

Sighting

Using an object either in the water or on shore to guide you and keep you on course during an open water swim is known as sighting. A boat, a marker buoy, a house or mountain on shore can all serve as things to "sight off of" and keep you on course during your open water swim. You need to determine these objects prior to your swim start. Many triathletes' swim times are slowed not by their technique or conditioning, but because they do not sight well and therefore do not swim in a straight line.

Sighting involves raising your head out of the water, and when you do this, your body position generally drops lower in the water, slowing you down. You therefore want to sight as infrequently as possible if your goal is to achieve a fast swim split. You will waste much more time however if you choose not to sight frequently and end up way off course, swimming much longer than the actual measured distance to compensate. So, ideally, you will sight just enough to keep yourself on course.

Although drafting on the bike may be illegal in many triathlons, drafting is not against the rules during the swim. Drafting during the swim entails following closely behind a swimmer, namely right on his or her toes, staying in that swimmer's "wake." This benefits you in two ways:

1. There is slightly decreased drag by swimming closely behind someone, and you therefore will save some energy.
2. Assuming that the person you are drafting off of stays on course and is swimming your

speed, you will not have to sight as often, keeping you more relaxed and preventing you from slowing down every time you raise your head. You can sight underwater on the person's body or even the bubbles he or she creates while swimming. Oftentimes the swimmer in front of you may slow down or speed up; this is not a problem. You simply then swim on and try to find someone else swimming at your speed, get behind him or her, and begin drafting once again.

So what's the solution to the challenges posed by the open water swim? Simple. You need to get acclimated to swimming in the open water and accustomed to sighting of off objects in the distance and swimmers in front of you. You can do this alone or with a friend or group of friends. Either an ocean or a lake will serve as a good place to practice your open water swimming.

A highly effective solution to dealing with the stress of open water swimming, both before the race and during, lies not in physical training but in mental training—relaxation exercises, self-talk, and visualization training. I will discuss these three techniques in the section on mental training.

 THE FLOATING BUOY

I participated in a Half-Ironman race that no longer exists; this may be due in part to the number of things that went wrong during the triathlons over the years. The swim was a mass start and entailed swimming a triangle (many swims are designed in this fashion)—out to a red buoy, turning left around the buoy and swimming downstream to another red buoy, then turning left again and swimming back to shore. Well, it just so happened that the second buoy came unhooked from its moorings and began to float slowly downstream. Many swimmers had already passed this marker and were on their way back to shore, but the slower swimmers continued to "chase" this buoy, not realizing that it was in fact moving! When race organizers finally realized that this had happened and the swimmers were not going to be able to "catch" this now moving target, they were forced to pick the remaining swimmers up in boats and bring them back to shore.

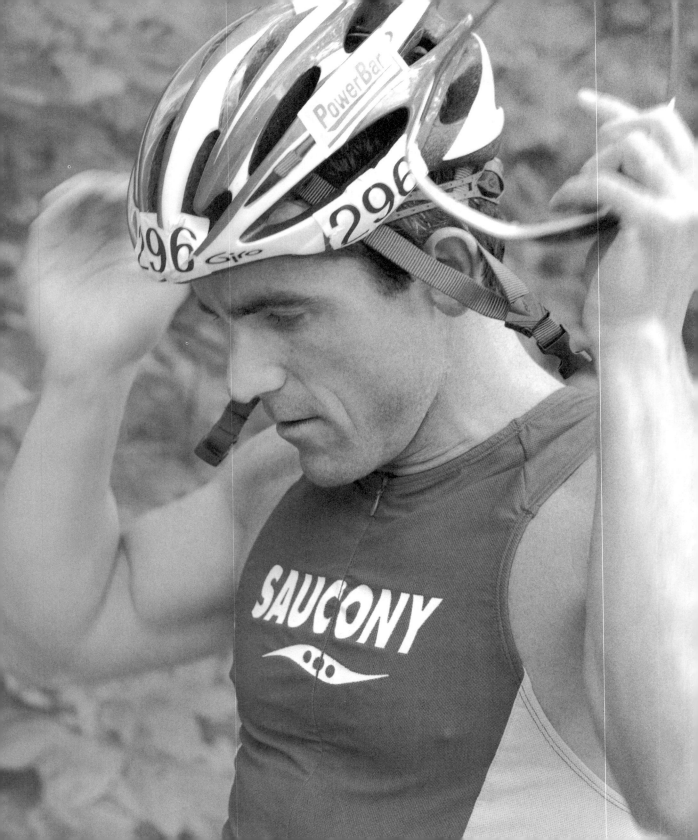

CHAPTER 7
Bike Training

"Time in the saddle," simply time spent riding your bike, is what it ultimately takes to really begin to improve your biking ability. It is no surprise that exceptional bikers such as Lance Armstrong have been riding since they were kids. It goes back to Specific Adaptations to Imposed Demands; that is, you get better at the motor skills that you practice. What many people fail to realize is that they get faster at swimming, biking, and running not from doing speed work per se, but by becoming more efficient at these disciplines, and this comes from sheer time spent just doing the activity. This is especially true of biking. Yes, speed work has its place, and I will outline several workouts that will indeed improve your bike splits, but it is time spent in the saddle that will really pay dividends to your bike performance as well as enjoyment of the sport.

BIKE WORKOUTS

One of the most frequently asked questions is "How can I be expected to ride at my goal pace on race day if I spend so much time riding more slowly?" The belief that you must ride fast all the time is what causes injury, burnout, and actual decreases in performance. Your slow days should be slow and your fast days should be fast, and you should spend little time in between, in what coaches refer to as the gray zone. You will do much of your training in the relatively "slow" zone, especially during the base phase of your training. Improvements in speed come through increased efficiency, judicious implementation of speed workouts, and, on race day, that unknown x-factor, "race-day magic." Go hard sometimes, go easy most of the time, and go home.

For those of you whose goal it is to simply finish your triathlon, you will bike by time and will not pay attention to specific bike workouts. You will indeed get faster, stronger, and build endurance by simply spending time on the bike. Bike distances will not be specified except for the Ironman program, where several 100-mile rides will be scheduled. For those of you who will be following the Performance program, we will utilize four different training zones for bike workouts. Each is based on perceived exertion in conjunction with relative speed.

1. *EZ: Easy effort.* Several miles per hour slower than your Race Pace goal. If none of these four zones is specified, then the intensity will always be EZ pace. The majority of your training will be done in this zone.

2. *RP: Race Pace.* Just as it sounds, the pace and perceived effort you wish to average for your specific race.

3. *JARP: Just Above Race Pace.* It should feel just above the effort you wish to maintain on race day.

4. **HE: Hard Effort.** Time-Trial-Type Intervals. These intervals are considerably above your Race Pace effort and speed. An example would be "2 × 5 minutes @ 2 minutes rest." This means that you would bike hard for five minutes, then recover while biking easy for two minutes, then bike hard for another five minutes.

You will also occasionally do hill repeat workouts to improve your biking strength. For example, a bike workout might specify a 1 hour bike with 4 hill repeats @ 30 minutes. This would mean that you would bike for 30 minutes, ending up at a hill that ideally takes you at least several minutes to climb. You then would climb up it hard, recover on the way down, repeat this four times, then bike back easy to cool down.

CADENCE

You will become a better biker by simply biking, by practicing the motor pattern over and over and over again. You will become more efficient, you will become stronger, and you will build up your endurance. One aspect of your cycling that you can pay attention to in order to improve your triathlon performance is your cadence, the rate at which you pedal. Many coaches now believe that you should try to maintain a high cadence as much as possible during the biking leg of the triathlon, and I support that theory. A high cadence will serve to save valuable energy while on the bike, but more importantly for triathletes, it will also "save" your legs for the run to follow. What you must never forget as a triathlete is, as pro triathlete and triathlon coach Troy Jacobson puts it so perfectly: *Triathlon is not about who goes the fastest, but who slows down the least.*

TRIATHLON VOCABULARY

Smaller Gears: Lower gears. Easier to turn the pedals. These are found on the smaller chain ring on the front and bigger chain rings on your back wheel.

Big Gear: Higher gears. Harder to turn the pedals. Generally found in the bigger chain ring on the front and smaller chain rings on your back wheel.

Mashing: Pushing a "big" gear while biking and pedaling against significant resistance at a slow cadence (revolutions per minute). Triathletes are often accused of utilizing this less-than-efficient style of biking by cyclists.

As a triathlete, you should try to practice maintaining a high cadence during your training rides. Pedaling in a big gear and pushing against more resistance will tire out most athletes' legs and leave them with "dead legs," legs that feel heavy and unable to hold a race pace for the run.

You may indeed post a faster bike split by riding in a bigger gear, but chances are this will cost you significantly more time in the end. There is no strict formula per se, but it seems that each minute pushed too hard on the bike translates into several minutes lost on the run. Do not forget that triathlon entails three sports and you will have to run after you bike. Push the bike too hard, and you will suffer on the run, possibly joining the ranks of the walkers who failed to adequately pace themselves during the bike leg.

As a triathlete, you should try to maintain a cadence of at least 85 RPMs (revolutions per minute) as much as possible while biking. Of course, you may not be able to maintain this cadence on steeper hills, but even then it is a good strategy to try to stay in the saddle and spin up them as much as possible. This takes practice but will pay dividends when it comes time to run. Does this strategy hold true for everyone? No. While maintaining a high cadence is a strategy utilized by many of the top triathletes and cyclists (Lance Armstrong for one), it all comes down to how fast you can go on the bike while preserving yourself for the run. If you can do this while pushing a big gear, then that is your technique. Just realize it does not seem to work for most come run time.

How do you know what your cadence is? Many bike computers come with cadence monitoring capabilities. You can also hold your hand out over one leg as you are pedaling and count how many times your knee comes up and hits your hand in fifteen seconds. Multiply this number by four and you have your cadence. Over time you should be able to go by feel and know your cadence pretty closely.

GROUP RIDES

Group rides are a great way to get your bike workouts in with company. They can also serve to help your speed and strength if you decide to ride with the faster groups. There is nothing that will make you go faster than your ego as you try to keep up with the faster riders, if that is your goal. Many group rides break up into smaller groups at the start by speed, such as A, B, and C groups, with A being the faster group out front and each successive group riding a little more slowly. You can ride with the slower group as your LSD, Long Slow Distance or EZ, rides if that is an appropriately slow pace. You can also ride with the faster groups as a modification of your speed work in your biking program. Just be careful that you do not spend all your time biking hard in group rides; this inevitably leads to injury, burnout, and decreased performance. Most towns have organized group rides; a great place to find out about them is through your local bike shop.

I like to take spin class. Count I count this as my bike workout?

I would say yes and no. If I told you that this was an acceptable substitution, you would be in for an unwelcome surprise come race day. The bottom line is that riding outside is different in several ways from riding indoors on a

TRIATHLON VOCABULARY

Getting dropped: This is what happens when you are riding with a group and cannot keep up the pace; you "get dropped," or fall behind. Unless there is a slower group behind you that catches up, often you end up riding home alone. This is a good incentive to push the pace and keep up with the group.

Pace line: The single-file line that emerges in group rides. In the pace line riders ride with their wheels several inches apart. Riders "draft" off of one another, using the rider in front of them as a type of wind shield to conserve their own energy. The leader, who is doing the most work because he has no one to break the wind for him, "pulls" or leads for a short duration, then moves to the left and allows the next rider in line to take the lead. He slowly lets the pace line pass him and gets back in as the last rider.

spin bike. There is no wind, no balance involved, your body position is different, most spin wheels are weighted and you can utilize this momentum to your advantage, and you control the tension. Use a spin bike when you simply cannot get outdoors due to weather, travel, et cetera, or when you need a change of pace. Do the majority of your training on a real bike. You get good at what you practice, so unless you are participating in an "indoor triathlon," get outside and ride!

When training on your bike, you should try to simulate your race-day conditions as much as possible, whenever possible. This means using the exact bike setup, nutrition, and clothing that you intend on using in the race. Too often, people ride one way for weeks and months in training and then make changes for their race without practicing with these changes. This can lead to major problems that you do not want to have to deal with during

your triathlon. Remember that you get accustomed to that with which you practice. Even the smallest change on race day can lead to disaster. Make sure that you have tried everything that pertains to the bike you intend on using on race day. This will not only help prevent unnecessary surprises, but will also give you increased confidence.

TRAINING IN INCLEMENT WEATHER

There are certain things we can control when it comes to triathlon and certain things that we cannot. True success comes as a result of realizing what we can manipulate and control and doing the work to do so. Conversely, and just as important, is to realize and accept that which we have no control over and let it go. Weather is one of these factors. We obviously have no say in what the weather will be like on race day. We cannot control the temperature, the wind, or the rain. What we can control is the experience of having trained in as many of these conditions as possible. The easiest way to do this is to stick to your program as closely as possible and not skip a workout due to the weather. Odds are such that most, if not all, of these conditions will arise at least once, if not several times, throughout your training. You will not have the luxury of staying inside and watching television on race day because it is raining or cold, so you might as well get used to working out at least once or twice in inclement weather, more often if you are following the Performance program. Many people skip workouts when there is bad weather, and these people will suffer both mentally and physically during their race as a consequence. I expect the weather on my race days to be rainy, windy, and cold; I am never disappointed, only pleasantly surprised. You should check the weather report before your triathlon to see what you need to wear, not to become depressed by a less-than-perfect weather report.

Of course safety comes first—do not ride, or run, for that matter, in conditions where your personal safety is compromised. Use common sense and skip the workout or train indoors when training outside becomes dangerous.

FIXING A FLAT

Many new bikers and triathletes do not know how to change a flat tire and therefore have one more thing to potentially worry about before as well as during a race. They often make it through training without getting a flat tire, and odds are their first flat will indeed happen at the most inopportune time. I have all of my clients learn to change a tire several times during their training so that they would be able to do so if it happened on race day. If you do not know how to change a tire, I recommend that you either go to a bike shop and learn there (many shops have seminars on just this topic) or have a triathlete or cyclist friend take you through the process. Of course, I could try to explain to you how it's done, but I find the explanation to be similar to describing swim drills; you really need to see it done in person to truly learn how to do it correctly.

There are two methods for inflating tires while on the road: bike pump and CO_2 cartridges. The bike pump, a modified version of the floor bike pump, is one that attaches right onto your bike frame or is carried in the pocket on the back of your bike jersey. CO_2 cartridges are small metal tubes filled with air. You purchase a special valve that has a hole to attach to the cartridge and another that fits onto the tire valve. You press the valve and the cartridge empties into the tube, inflating it.

Both methods work equally well, so why should you choose one over the other? Realize first that you can run out of CO_2s, but the bike pump will always provide you with air. Once you buy the pump, that's it; CO_2s, on the other hand, need to be replaced. The bike pump weighs more than the CO_2s, however, and for those athletes who are trying to minimize the weight of the bike, CO_2s are the better choice. There are also those who do not want to attach the pump to their frame or deal with having it on their backs during rides, so they choose CO_2s as well. If speed and weight are not your concern and piece of mind is, then I would recommend attaching a bike pump to your frame. You can purchase very small pumps that will fill your flats for many hundreds of training miles ridden.

WHAT TO BRING ON TRAINING RIDES

Here are is list of items that you will want to consider bringing with you on training rides.

1. *Spare tubes:* I recommend at least two in case of multiple flat tires.
2. *Money:* For pit stops to get additional drinks and food on longer rides, as well as for emergencies.
3. *A credit card:* For bigger emergencies. You never know what you may need and when you may need it, and the cash you have with you may not be enough to cover it.
4. *A bike pump or CO2 cartridges:* To fill those inevitable flat tires.
5. *Tire levers:* To help you change the tubes on your clinchers.
6. *A multifunction bike tool:* For tightening screws and performing bike adjustments when necessary.
7. *A cell phone:* For emergencies.

There are numerous methods for carrying these items during training rides. Again, what you choose depends upon your specific bike setup and personal preference. Attaching a bike bag underneath your seat is a common way to carry all your extra gear.

1. *Fanny pack:* This is my preferred method for training rides. I have a small pack around my waist filled with all the necessary items. It is light and comfortable and I do not notice I am wearing it.
2. *Bike jersey pockets:* Some riders prefer to stuff the pockets found in the back of most bike jerseys with their gear. I personally find this to be uncomfortable, especially when you are carrying all of the items outlined above.

3. *Bike bags:* Small bags that usually attach under your seat but can also attach to your top tube or in between your aerobars. This is a popular method as you simply fill the bag with all your necessities and they are there when you need them—you don't have to remember to bring them with you for each ride.
4. *Bike bottle:* Necessity is the mother of invention, and triathletes are no exception to this rule. Some athletes use a bike bottle with the top off or cut off to hold their bike gear. They usually will use one of the two bike cages behind them for this "gear bottle." Just be aware that you have to pack this bottle carefully, as one hole in the road or bump can send all of the contents flying.

HYDRATION ON THE BIKE

Taking in fluids on the bike is a necessity and becomes more important as the length of your training rides and triathlon race distances increase. Dehydration is a common cause of decreased race performance and will be discussed in greater detail in the chapter on nutrition. What you need to decide is what method you will use to carry your fluids on the bike, as there are several to choose from. Again, you can choose to use more than one method for fluid replacement:

1. Aerobar bike bottle
2. Bike bottle cage on the seat tube
3. Bike bottle cage on the down tube
4. Bike bottles cages behind the seat (choice of 1 or 2)
5. CamelBak system

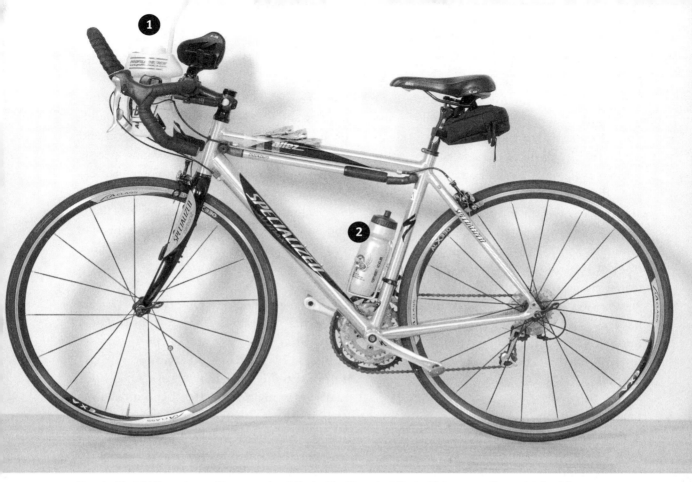

Two-bottle tri-bike set-up with an aerobar bike bottle (1) and a bike bottle cage on the seat tube (2).

Bike Bottle Cages

Certain styles of bike will determine where you can and cannot carry fluids. For example, my Aegis Trident has a flat down tube that is not able to have a bike bottle cage mounted to it. Softride bikes have no seat tubes, so you have to mount the bottle cages on the down tube or behind the seat. If you choose to use bike bottles, I recommend that you attach at least two, even for those of you who will be racing sprint triathlons exclusively. I use one on my seat tube and two attached behind my seat. I have experimented with the aerobar bottle and found that I prefer to use bottles that I can take out and hold while I ride.

The Aerobar Bike Bottle

This is a specially shaped bottle that attaches between your aerobars and remains there. It has a straw that sticks up out of it, which you sip from while leaning over or while in the aero position. It also comes with a piece of netting that stays inside the bottle and keeps the fluids from splashing out as you ride over rougher surfaces. During a race, you take a bottle at the aid station, pour it into the aerobar bottle, and throw the empty bottle back to the aid station volunteers. (I will discuss the aid stations in greater detail in the chapter on racing.) One of the advantages of the aerobar system is that the bottle is in front of you, directly in your line of sight. It may seem trivial, but during a race, many people "forget" to drink their fluids on a regular schedule, and by having the bottle directly in front of you, you are constantly reminded to drink. Some people find drinking from the aerobar system easier, while others find it harder. It definitely takes practice to take the bottle from the aid station volunteer, open it, dump it into the aerobar bottle, and discard the empty bottle.

CamelBak System

The CamelBak is a brand name for a hydration system that you wear on your back like a backpack. Essentially a bladder with shoulder straps, it comes in various sizes and styles and has a strawlike tube that you sip from. The CamelBak is used less frequently by triathletes than bike bottles are, but some do prefer getting their liquids by this method while training as well as racing.

Can I use a CamelBak during my training rides and bike bottles during the race?

Yes, but I would recommend that you try to get your fluids the same way while training that you do during racing. The closer your training rides simulate racing, the better. For example, I try to take in one bottle of Gatorade every 30

minutes on the bike. I know exactly how many calories are in each bottle, and how these calories add up along with my other nutrition on the bike. If I were to use a CamelBak while training and bike bottles while racing, I wouldn't have tested this fluid intake program and this would complicate issues. Many people experience cramping and gastrointestinal distress during triathlons due to underfueling, overfueling, or switching to new forms of fluids and nutrition—the key is to train with the plan you intend to follow while racing to minimize the chances of these occurrences.

Okay, I'm going to train with three bike bottles and drink one every half hour. What do I do if I am riding for three hours? I can't carry six bottles, so I'll be three bottles short.

I deal with this issue in two ways. One, I primarily plan my rides so that I end up at a gas station or convenience store at the exact time I need to refuel. If that is not an option and you are riding a few loop courses close to home, you can always hide bottles along the way before your ride or end up back at home, refuel, then finish your ride. Do not make a habit of riding long distances without the proper liquids and nutrition; your rides will suffer, your recovery will suffer, and you will not have "rehearsed" this important aspect of your training come race day.

So, it is up to you to decide how you plan on carrying your fluids with you while you bike. There have been studies about which method is most aerodynamic, but for most people's purposes, I find that to be the least important factor when deciding on what type of system to use. What is most important is choosing a method that you will use; in other words, one that encourages you to drink at regular intervals. It doesn't matter how aerodynamic your bike is if you are dehydrated.

NUTRITION ON THE BIKE

For those of you competing in longer-distance triathlons, you will need to take in more calories while on the bike to fuel your bike as well as your run. Nutrition can be broken down into liquids, semisolids, and solids. Which you choose is highly individualized and takes experimentation during your practice rides. I will discuss fuel in greater detail in the chapter on nutrition, but first I will illustrate several methods that you can use to carry the nutrition while on the bike.

Why do I need to carry nutrition with me during the race? My Half-Ironman race information packet says they will have aid stations every ten miles—Gatorade, energy bars, bananas, water—why can't I just get everything along the way?

Many races do have fully stocked aid stations on both the bike and the run, especially Ironman races. While you will indeed get liquids as well as food from these stations, there are several important reasons why you need to bring calories with you as well.

1. Ten miles is not a short distance—roughly thirty minutes of biking, depending on the rider and the course. You will want to have taken in calories before you arrive at the first aid station.
2. Each race has different types, brands, and flavors of nutrition. This is especially true

if you plan on traveling to races, particularly international races. Unless you have practiced with what they will be providing on the course, the nutrition provided may not "work" for you and could potentially cause you gastrointestinal distress. You also should have a good idea of how many calories you will be taking in each hour, and you may not know the caloric content of the nutrition provided.

3. Aid stations can run out of certain items. If you were desperately hoping to get a Power-Bar at your next aid station and they did not have one, you would now have 30 more minutes to go without those calories. You should be on a specific eating and drinking schedule, and the aid stations might not have what you need when you need it.

You generally want to take in the majority of your calories in liquid or semisolid form, but again, this is highly individualistic and takes experimentation to discover what works best for you. As you experiment, here are several different methods of "carrying calories" with you on the bike:

1. *Water bottles/aerobottle/CamelBak:* All of the ways in which you carry your liquids are potential methods you can utilize to carry your liquid calories as well. Fluids like Gatorade and PowerBar Performance have calories and carbohydrates in them and can be part of your strategy. More calorically dense liquids such as meal replacements like Ensure (my preferred method of taking in the majority of my calories while on the bike) can also be held in your fluid containers.

2. *Bike jersey pockets:* Once again, those pockets in the back of your bike jersey can be used to hold some of your nutrition such as bars or gels. (Now you can see why you need to find several ways to carry items with you on the bike; if you have already decided to carry your spare tubes, tool, and bike pump in your pockets, then adding your food in as well might be a little bit much!)

3. *Bike bags:* There are specially designed bags that attach in different ways to your top tube as well as to your handlebars and seat post. You can store your gels, bars, even a peanut-butter-and-jelly sandwich in here and have relatively easy access to them as you ride.

4. *Gel flask:* There are plastic flasks that attach to your bike frame that you can fill with your gel nutrition. The flask has Velcro on it, which holds it in place until you need it. This is a convenient method to take in semi-solids as you don't have to open the packets while you ride. Each flask holds multiple gels and therefore can provide several hundred calories to your overall intake.

5. *Your top tube:* Again, necessity is the mother of invention, and this is evidenced by how some triathletes carry nutrition on the top tube of their bike. Don't have a gel flask but want to carry your gels on your top tube? No problem—all you need is some tape. You begin by taping just the top of the first gel packet to your top tube close to your handlebars. You then tape the next one underneath the first the same way, so that the first lies on top of the second. You continue taping your gels in this manner until you have all

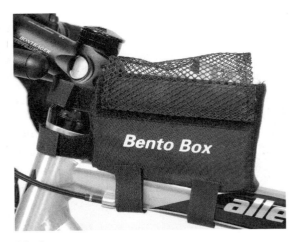
Bike bag

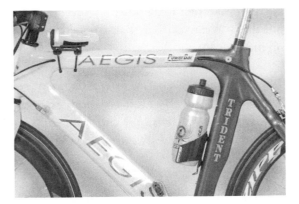
Gel flask

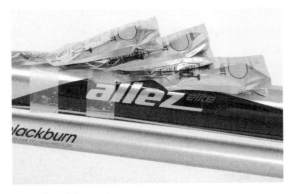
Top tube with snacks

your gels on the top tube. Then, during the race you will tear off the first gel, opening it in the process as you have taped the top down. The key is to get it to your mouth and empty the contents as fast as possible—if you take too long, you could be covered with strings of sticky gel for the remainder of the race. Obviously, this takes some practice, and you should absolutely try it on training rides first.

6. *Fanny pack:* Worn like a belt around your waist with the pack behind you, a fanny pack can be stuffed with almost all of the items you may need for your triathlon. Gels, bars, spare tubes, tire levers, and bike tool can all fit in and can be accessed during riding by spinning the bag around to your front or when stopped completely.

CHAFING

Sitting on a bike seat for prolonged periods of time can bring about some uncomfortable chafing issues, especially in the upper quads between your legs. After your first long workout, you will find out where your personal problem areas lie the moment the water hits your body when you take a shower. People used to use Vaseline or similar products to prevent these uncomfortable rashes; now they have specific products on the market for these unique athletic chafing issues. I highly recommend and use Body Glide—unlike Vaseline, you can't feel it on you, yet it does a great job of preventing rashes and burns. It comes packaged like a roll-on deodorant, and before your bike workouts, you merely spread it on those body parts that have a tendency to chafe.

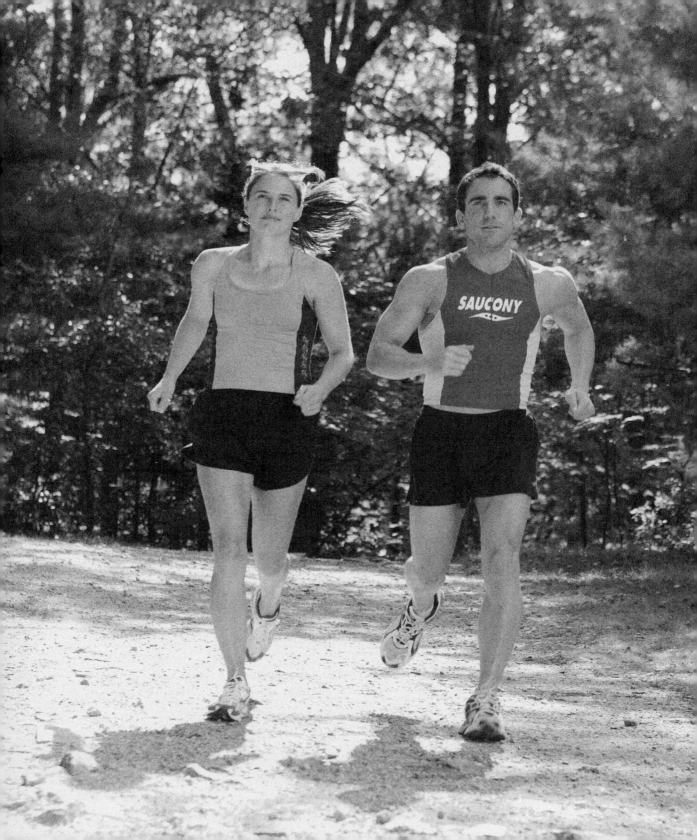

CHAPTER 8
Run Training

Running is my personal favorite of the three triathlon disciplines. I love the sheer simplicity of running; all you really need to do it is a good pair of sneakers. You can do it almost anywhere as well. One aspect of travel that I enjoy immensely is running wherever I am—lacing on a pair of running shoes and exploring the unknown by foot. I believe deeply that we have set the bar incredibly low when it comes to fitness and especially running; so many people are missing out on the innumerable benefits, both physically and mentally, that come from running. In my fitness consulting for the media, I am often asked what the "best" exercise to lose weight is, and my reply is always running. When I am asked what the "best" exercise is to get great abdominals, my answer is running as well.

For those of you whose goal it is to finish your first triathlon, you will simply run as part of your program. There will be no special instructions other than the time specified for each workout that you will run. However, for the Half-Ironman and Ironman programs, there will be a few runs where mileage is specified.

Why aren't all the run workouts done by miles? Why run by time?
One of the main reasons I design runs by time is so that you can have the freedom to run wherever you wish, whenever you wish. You can run out the door and choose whatever route you want, vary it as you go, and change it day to day if you so choose. This also makes running while traveling significantly easier; you don't have to spend any time with a local map figuring out distances; you can just run. You also don't need to waste time after a run in your car measuring out the distance of the run you just completed. That time can be better spent stretching! Remember how strongly I feel that consistency of your workouts is one of the major secrets to success; by allowing you to vary your run courses, you will stay mentally fresh, you will vary the difficulty of your workouts, and you will help prevent burnout.

For the longer-distance triathletes doing Half-Ironman- and Ironman-distance races, you will have a few runs where mileage is specified to ensure that you have run the longer distances. I believe that this is confidence building and that there is psychological value in knowing that you have run close to your race distance in training.

Similar to biking, you will get faster, stronger, and build endurance by simply logging miles while running. For those following the Performance Program, you will have speed elements judiciously added to your schedules. It has been my experience that speed workouts, especially at the track, are where so many runners and triathletes injure themselves. Speed workouts should be done:

1. After building a significant base of strength
2. Progressively; you shouldn't begin with 12-mile repeats
3. After an adequate warm-up
4. And, followed by an adequate cool-down
5. With at least one easy workout following the speed workout, preferably two

It would be very easy for me to design these programs with a great deal of hard and complex speed training involved. I have read many books and know of many coaches who prescribe such workouts and, again, I have found many of the athletes who attempt to follow these programs end up injured, often for long periods of time. In my opinion, intensity needs to be implemented sparingly and only when preceded by base-building consistency.

For those following the Performance Program, you will utilize the same four intensities for running as for biking:

1. *EZ: Easy runs.* These are 1 to 2 minutes slower than your Race Pace goal. Easy effort. The majority of your training will be done at this effort.
2. *RP: Race Pace.* Just as it sounds, the pace and perceived effort are what you wish to average for your specific race.
3. *JARP: Just Above Race Pace.* It should feel just above the effort you wish to maintain on race day.
4. *HE: Hard Effort.* These intervals are considerably above your Race Pace effort and speed. An example would be "2 x 3 minutes @ 1 minute rest." This means

that you would run hard for three minutes, then recover while jogging easy for one minute, then run hard for another three minutes.

When should I replace my running shoes?

Sooner rather than later. I recommend changing them every 300 to 500 miles. It may cost a little more to replace them this frequently, but running in old, worn-down shoes can cause numerous different running injuries. The money spent on new shoes will be saved on physical therapy visits caused by logging too many mile in the same shoes. My rule of thumb: If your running shoes look old, you have been running in them way too long. Most likely your shoes will not look like they need to be replaced at the 300- to 500-mile mark unless you have had several workouts in inclement weather.

Can I do my run workouts on the treadmill?

Yes and no. Running on the treadmill is not exactly like running outside, and there are actually both pros and cons associated with training on a treadmill. The bottom line is that you will not be doing your triathlon run on a treadmill (I hope!), so you want to get used to running outdoors as much as possible. Nasty weather may be a reason to run on the treadmill, but remember that you may have this type of weather on race day, so you do want to train in it occasionally, if possible. You may also use the treadmill when you are traveling and unable to run outside. The treadmill can actually be a good training tool for occasional workouts where you will be running at a specific pace and therefore you can program it to whatever pace you wish. I also believe that running on a treadmill can be good mental training due to the sheer monotony of running in place like a hamster. You will definitely strengthen your mind while enduring long treadmill sessions. Short answer? Do the majority of your training outside and use the treadmill occasionally.

There will also be track workouts for those of you following the Performance Program. These workouts will specify "repeats" of laps around a standard running track:

- 400s—One lap
- 800s—Two laps
- Miles—Four laps

The goal of repeats is to run them hard, considerably above Race Pace, building speed as you go and finishing each one a little faster than you started. You must warm up before performing these repeats, by running easy for one to two miles. You need not do the warm-up on the track itself; you can run out on roads or trails nearby and end up at the track after a few miles. Likewise, you need to cool down in the same manner in which you warmed up. Run easy for one to two miles after performing your repeats, to help work the lactic acid through your system.

RUNNING FORM

There are many schools of thought concerning what is considered to be the "best" running form. I believe that while there are guidelines that you should consider while examining and perfecting your running style, each person does have a "personal" running style. The bottom line is, does your form allow you to go fast and far without causing you injury? Just as one person's aero position may not work for you, another's running style may not, either. Whenever I think of running form and exceptions to the rules, I think of the elite female marathoner who runs with her arms hanging straight down at her sides. No arm swing, just both arms

TRIATHLON VOCABULARY

Running economy: Namely "how" you run. While individual differences do exist, there is such a thing as "good running form." Great runners require less energy to perform at high speeds, and part of this has to do with the manner in which they run. Speed training not only improves overall speed by making physiological changes to your body, but it also forces you to become a more economical runner, making you faster as a result. I also believe that running long distances over time also forces us to become more economical runners. Our bodies are incredibly smart machines, and as we get more and more fatigued during a long run, we simply cannot afford to waste energy and our body adapts in order to survive. Chances are you won't see someone running with too much bounce at mile 22 of a marathon.

hanging lifelessly at her sides. It's tough to criticize her form as she runs world-class times in the marathon. Consider the following basics when working on improving your running economy, refining and defining your own personal running style:

1. Arms bent to roughly 90 degrees
2. Arm swing front to back, not side to side
3. Initiating your arm swing from your shoulders
4. Hands gently cupped
5. Shoulders down and back
6. Soft foot strike
7. Relax, relax, relax!

Relax your entire body from your head right down through to your toes. Have you ever watched the face of an Olympic sprinter in slow motion? Their cheeks flap wildly because these runners have learned to relax all of their muscles, including the smallest muscles of their face. The bottom line is that the more relaxed you are, the more you will improve your running economy. The more you are able to improve your running economy, the less energy you will expend at higher intensities, and the faster you will run.

CHAFING ISSUES

Like biking, running also has its chafing issues, only there seem to be a few more spots that tend to get tender while running than biking. The solution is the same, rubbing a product like Body Glide on these areas before your run workouts. Spots may include but are not limited to: between your upper legs, under your arms near your armpits where your arms will rub against your body, nipples and the groin area for men, and for women, on the breastbone where running bras will rub. Chafing tends to be more of an issue the longer your workouts are, but you should get in the habit of protecting yourself with a little product before all workouts.

CARRYING FLUIDS AND NUTRITION

One of the more difficult things to do during run training is to get in adequate fluids and calories, especially during longer runs. Most people do these workouts in a perpetual state of dehydration and on the verge of "bonking." Yes, you can get through these runs with no fluids or nutrition, but this will result in less-than-optimal workouts and longer recovery times afterward. Remember, train like you will race.

There are several ways to deal with this issue; here are three that I recommend:

1. *The Fuel Belt:* Over the years, they have invented better and better belt systems with which to carry fluids and liquid nutrition while you run. My favorite, and the more popular brand used by triathletes and runners, is the Fuel Belt. There are many different styles to choose from, with varying numbers of bottles and small Velcro pockets to hold items such as salt tablets. I recommend wearing one for all runs lasting forty-five minutes or more. You will get accustomed to having it on as well as practice taking in fluids, both of which will benefit you during your workouts as well as on race day.

2. *Leave fluids and nutrition along your course:* Drive your running route the day before your longer runs and stash your food and drinks every several miles or so.

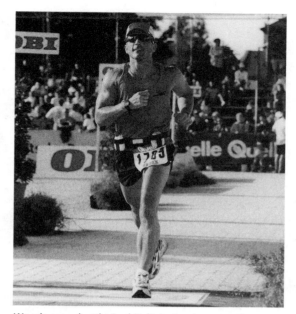

Wearing a 4-bottle Fuel Belt during Ironman Germany

3. *Bring money:* Carry cash with you and time your run so that you end up at a convenience store or gas station every twenty to thirty minutes to refuel.

I hurt my knee while running. Should I put ice on it or heat?

The general rule is to use ice for the first twenty-four to forty-eight hours immediately following an injury, to reduce the swelling and slow down the inflammation process. The ice will help to constrict the blood vessels in the affected area and reduce the inflammatory response. Place ice on the area for ten to fifteen minutes; then remove it for ten to fifteen minutes. Repeat this several times throughout the day, and try to get the ice on the injured area as soon as possible following the event. Of course, if the injury is great, then you should have it checked out by a sports doctor.

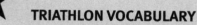

★ TRIATHLON VOCABULARY

Bonk: Quite simply, to run out of gas during your race; usually occurring on the run. Symptoms may include (but are not limited to!) being lightheaded, dizzy, and having legs that feel like lead. Some say that it is the result of running out of glycogen stores, some say it is from the lack of adequate endurance training, and others contend that it is a combination of the two. Quite often it happens at around mile 20 of a marathon, and for a good scientific reason if you haven't adequately fueled yourself.

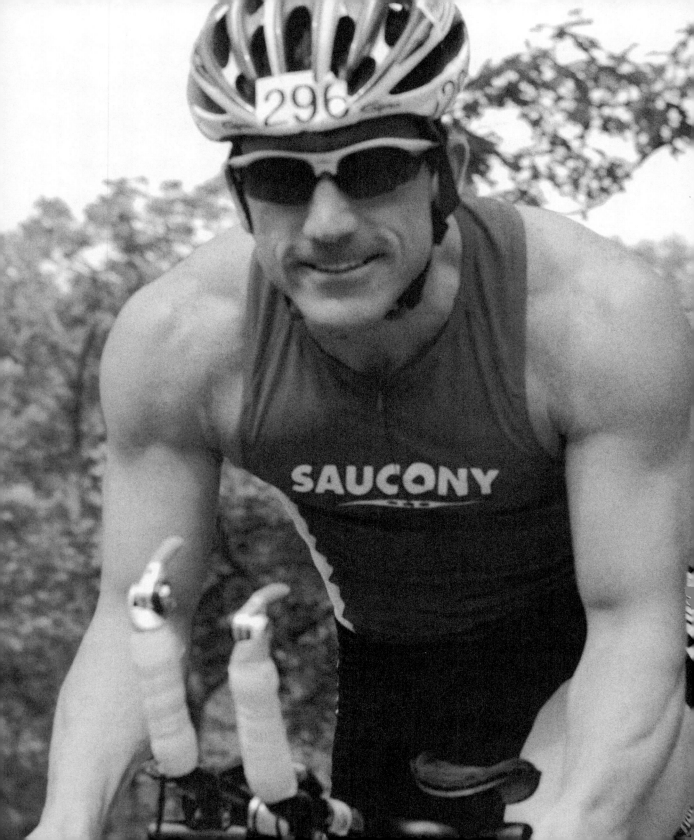

CHAPTER 9
Triathlon Training

So now you have assembled the basic equipment necessary or perhaps you have splurged and bought a high-end bike and a handful of fun triathlon toys and accessories. Whichever the case, now it's time to do the work, to train. I will repeat these words over and over again because I think it is so crucial in this sport: It's not about the equipment. It's about time spent in the pool, on the bike, and pounding the pavement in those running shoes. And it's not necessarily about how long you spend doing any of these three disciplines, either. It's about *quality* training, not *quantity*. An hour of swimming poorly in the pool only serves to reinforce bad swim technique, whereas thirty minutes of quality drill work will improve your stroke, lowering your swim split and adding to your race-day enjoyment as well.

THE 12-WEEK PLAN

Each 12-week plan will consist of the same framework and periodization model. What is periodization? Simply put, it is a method of gradually increasing your training over time, then decreasing the training for a short time, then building back up again. It is one of the major secrets to true triathlon success. Most people work out the same way each week, and this is far from the optimal way to train. It eventually leads to potential injury, overtraining, and diminished performances. The goal is to stress

the body, then let it recover, then stress it a little further, then let it recover again, repeating this several times and then recovering in preparation for the race. For those people who do increase their training over time, many do not include the "down week" or recovery week, and this, too, leads to the same negative results previously described.

Periodization involves three cycles: the macrocycle, mesocycle, and microcycle. All smart athletes now use this framework—runners, football players, hockey players, any athlete who prepares in the off-season and builds gradually up to his or her season. These cycles can vary in length, depending on numerous factors, not the least of which is the coach's training philosophy. I have designed the 12-week triathlon training plans utilizing the following periodization model.

Macrocycle: The macrocycle is the entire training plan, for our purposes, twelve weeks long.

Mesocycle: These are the training blocks that comprise the macrocycle. We will be using four mesocycles: the Base, Build, Peak, and Taper Phases. Within these phases will be three weeks of gradually increasing volume of training, followed by one week of sharply reduced training. This "down week" is when the body recovers and rebuilds from the previous weeks of training and prepares itself for the block to come. Next comes the Peak Phase, two weeks of the highest training volume to "peak" you for your triathlon. Last comes the Taper Phase, two weeks of gradually reduced volume to "absorb" the prior ten weeks of training, allowing your body to recover fully so that it will be ready to go on race day.

Microcycle: Our microcycles consist of one week of training, starting on Monday and ending on Sunday. The mesocycles are made up of several microcycles. All 12-week programs entail a Base mesocycle comprised of four microcycles, a Build mesocycle comprised of four microcycles, a Peak mesocycle that is two microcycles long, and a two–microcycle-long Taper mesocycle.

HEART RATE ZONES

Wearing heart rate monitors and training with heart rate zones have become increasingly more popular over the past decade. Everyone seems to have a heart rate monitor now—spin classes are filled with pedalers from weekend warriors to housewives, all sporting the newest monitor and watching the rise and fall of their heart rates during their workouts. Article after article is written about training by heart rate, and training intensities are defined as narrowly as within several percentage points.

12-*Week Triathlete Periodized Training Plan*

WEEK	Mon	Tues	Wed	Thurs	Fri	Sat	Sun
BASE PHASE							
12							
11							
10							
9							
BUILD PHASE							
8							
7							
6							
PEAK PHASE							
5							
4							
3							
TAPER PHASE							
2							
1							

What hasn't changed is the complexity of training by heart rate zones. Determining accurate individual training zones is much more difficult than most people realize, and this is compounded when you try to determine the appropriate zones for swimming, biking, and running. Add in the fluctuations in heart rate due to such factors as environmental conditions and sickness and the relative ranges of these heart rate zones are further compromised.

It has been my experience that the vast majority of triathletes need not train by heart rate zones to perform at a high level. While using a heart rate monitor can be an effective training aid when used in conjunction with perceived exertion and performance times, I believe that triathletes need to focus more on the consistency of their workouts rather than heart rate readings. Too many triathletes spend too much time focused on the gadgets and the gear rather than simply getting out and getting into their workouts. It is because of this belief that I designed the intensity of the Performance training plans based on the following four zones: EZ (Easy), RP (Race Pace), JARP (Just above Race Pace), and HE (Hard Effort). I believe that these four intensities are integral to improving performance and are best achieved by matching "feel" with speed and time, not heart rate zones.

TRIATHLON TRAINING PROGRAMS

In each of the following programs, you'll notice that there are two final weeks, or "Week 1s," outlined. This is because some of your triathlons will take place on Saturday and others on Sunday—simply choose the final Taper week according to your specific race day.

TRAINING PROGRAM NOTES

1. When no intensity is specified, you should run and/or bike at a comfortable pace—"EZ."

2. Tuesday runs for Performance plans can be done either on the track or on the road.

3. "4x400s @ 30 sec rest." This type of Tuesday run speed workout means you will run a 400 at a Hard Effort, jog easy for 30 seconds, then repeat this three more times. This goes for 800s and mile repeats as well. For example, "4x1 mi @ 2 min rest" means that you will run one mile at a Hard Effort, jog easy for 2 minutes, then repeat this progression three more times.

4. All run speed workouts must begin with a 1- to 2-mile easy warm-up jog and be followed by a 1- to 2-mile cool-down jog.

5. Bike workouts such as "60 min w/20 min JARP Then 30 min JARP" mean that you will bike at a comfortable pace for the first 40 minutes, then bike Just Above Race Pace for the final 20 minutes, then run for 30 minutes Just Above Race Pace immediately following the bike.

6. "2 hr w/3x5 min HE @ 2 min rest": During this type of bike workout, you will bike comfortably for the first half of the workout, then bike at a Hard Effort for 5 minutes, bike easy again for 2 minutes to recover, repeat this two more times, then bike easy for the remainder of the workout.

7. You should always begin at an easy pace to warm up before performing an interval with an increased intensity, as well as leave yourself time to cool down. So, for a run workout such as "60 min w/15 min JARP," you should warm up at an easy pace for about 30 minutes, then run Just Above Race Pace for 15 minutes, then cool down at an easy pace for the remaining 15 minutes.

BRICK WORKOUTS

"Brick" workouts are the ones with a bike time followed by "then" and a run time. So, you will bike and then run immediately after. These workouts will help you get used to running after biking so that you don't feel like a penguin waddling along during the final leg of your triathlon. Ideally, you will do your bike workout then run almost immediately after, taking really no more than five minutes to change from the bike to the run. At first, trying to run so soon after your bike session will feel incredibly strange. You will feel really sluggish and your legs will undoubtedly feel like two sticks of lead. This is normal. Over time, you will be amazed at how you will feel better and better while running during your brick workouts.

I believe that the brick workout is essential to your performance as a triathlete. If you had to choose one workout to do on the weekend, choose the brick. The ability to run effectively after biking is not easy. The number of people who end up walking during the run of longer-distance triathlons is a testament to this fact.

Can I do an occasional brick workout at the gym, biking on a spin bike or stationary bike and then running on the treadmill?
Sure. This type of workout will also help you become more accustomed to running after biking. Just remember that biking and running

indoors is not quite the same as biking and running outdoors. Unless your triathlon will take place on stationary bikes and treadmills, be sure to do most of your training outdoors.

MASSAGE

I think triathlon training gives us a perfect reason to justify getting massages. When we train hard, we inevitably get sore, and one good way to loosen up those muscles and work out those knots is a good massage. While there are many claims about the supposed benefits of massage that I may question, I do believe that massage is extremely beneficial to athletes in general and triathletes in particular. It will loosen up muscles that become irritated, tight, and sore from training, such as the shoulders and upper back from swimming; the upper and lower back from biking, especially in the aero position; and, of course, the legs from both biking and running. I believe that massage prevents possible future injuries by working out these muscular issues, helping to rehabilitate repetitive stress injuries as well as correcting abnormalities caused by training that may force you to adjust your technique in any of the three disciplines and present problems elsewhere as a result. It's smart to be proactive rather than reactive as well; start getting massages before you have muscular issues, to prevent them rather than fix them. How often you get a massage essentially comes down to how much you are willing to spend on them. Many clubs sell packages of 5 or 10; once a week is great, especially on your off-day to recover. Getting a massage once every two weeks or once a month will also provide benefits. Remember, it's about working hard and recovering well.

Foam Rollers

Foam rollers, those white Styrofoam logs you may have seen in your gym or in a physical therapist's office, are simple yet extremely effective pieces of fitness equipment. They have many uses, including self-massage and stretching. You simply "roll" over them to massage and stretch sore and tight muscles. I use them for my quadriceps and especially for my iliotibial (IT) bands. The IT band is a thick band of tissue that runs along the outside of your legs from your hips down to your knees. When they are tight, they can cause pain in the outside of your knees, and triathlon training can definitely cause tightness in your IT bands. To stretch them with the roller, you simply lie on your side with it under the side of your thigh, then roll it up to your hip and back down to your knee, using your body weight to massage the area. This is a simple yet extremely effective way of preventing, as well as curing, IT band syndrome.

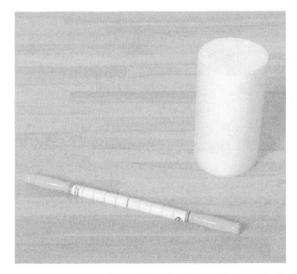

These two items, The Stick and a foam roller, are both great tools to use for self-massage.

Another simple yet extremely effective tool for self-massage is The Stick. After workouts, just run The Stick up and down your quadriceps, hamstrings, and calves for thirty seconds or so.

YOUR JOURNAL

At the end of this book are two journals for you to write down the particulars of your daily triathlon workouts as well as your strength training workouts. Use them. I have included them right in this book so that you will be more likely to keep track of your training. Do it and do it consistently. It will make a world of difference. We are all experiments of one when it comes to our triathlon training, and you must discover your individuality through trial and error, attempting to determine cause and effect and make changes for the better. Keeping notes on your training will allow you to slowly uncover what works and does not work for you. If a particular injury appears, you can look back at your notes and see if you can determine the potential cause by examining the specifics of your training. Feel lightheaded after a long bike ride? Note what you brought along as nutrition and hydration and modify it for the next similar workout. Stomachache after drinking a certain carbohydrate drink while on the bike? Make a note of it and try a different brand next time. It may sound goofy, but it is absolutely true; your workouts are all small "experiments" whereby you are attempting to come up with the recipes that bring about your best performances. Your notes need not and should not be complex. I purposely made the charts as simple as possible so that you can tailor them to whatever information you think is noteworthy that day. Be sure to include the basics and then add in anything new you might have tried or anything that happened during the workout that may be noteworthy. These journals will serve several functions as well. We often have poor or selective memories when it comes to what we actually did or did not do in our training, and these records will serve as the judge and jury. They will indicate whether or not you have been skipping too many workouts or have been overtraining, they will illustrate your progress in all three sports as well as in the weight room, and they will serve as an incredible confidence builder when you reread them all in the days leading up to your triathlon and see how hard you have worked, how ready you are for your race.

INJURIES

As with any exercise program, triathlon training will undoubtedly come with a few aches and pains, as well as potential injuries. So you need to determine the difference between soreness and pain. It is okay to train when sore, but it is not advisable to "work through" pain. That only leads to making the injury worse and potentially having to stop training for an extended period of time.

There is a difference between soreness and pain, and being sore is natural, especially at the beginning of your training as your body adapts to this new level of activity. In my opinion, too many people use soreness as an excuse not to exercise, using sore knees or muscles as a way out of taking care of their bodies. Given this same logic, people would stop eating ice cream or pizza the first time they experienced an "ice cream headache" or burned their mouths on hot pizza. Use your body and you will undoubtedly feel it; over time, you will grow stronger and fitter and healthier as a result. Be aware that some soreness may never go away completely if you continue to challenge your body; this is what I refer to as a "good soreness" and is not the same feeling you experience when you start a new training program.

So, don't quit training just because you are sore. Many people argue that an activity like running is bad for you, but inactivity is the real danger. Running does not cause injury per se, but rather illuminates weaknesses and imbalances in your body that need to be addressed. Without running you may not realize these issues and would not be forced to correct them, and they would present much bigger problems further down the road.

The key to dealing with real injuries and pain is to deal with them immediately. I could provide you with a lengthy discussion of injuries, their symptoms as well as their causes, and you could attempt to self-diagnose your pain, but that job is much better left to professional sports doctors. You should find a highly qualified sports doctor in your area and use him or her as part as your overall training plan. Pain will inevitably occur, but the sooner you deal with it, and the smarter you go about fixing the issue, the less likely you are to be injured in the future.

I am not half as proud of the high number, frequency, and length of endurance races that I compete in as much as I am that I do so while being injury-free. This comes in large part to consistency of training in all departments: swimming, biking, running, strength training, stretching, and a healthy diet. Do any one thing to excess, and problems will inevitably arise. Running is not bad for you; running exclusively, without strength training, cross training, and stretching, is.

To help you be proactive and prevent possible injury, here is a list of some of the common causes of triathlon-related injuries:

1. Doing too much too soon
2. Muscle weaknesses
3. Muscle imbalances
4. Flexibility issues—tight muscles
5. Wearing improper running shoes
6. Improper bike-seat height—too high or too low
7. Running frequently on the same side of a sloped road
8. Individual biomechanical issues like leg-length discrepancies and high or flat arches.

One of the most common causes of injury is doing too much, too soon. This is why it is so important that you follow a periodized plan and build up slowly. You cannot cram workouts in if you miss them, and you should not lengthen workouts just because you feel good that day.

The good news is that all of the above-mentioned issues can be corrected. What you need to do is cease training immediately when you feel true pain and seek the advice of a sports medicine professional. Taking two, three, or seven days off to deal with an issue is much smarter than having an injury plague you for months, if not longer, and force you to stop training altogether and perhaps even miss your race.

Sprint Distance Program

Sprint Distance Program—Finish

Week	Day	Weights	Swim	Bike	Run
BASE PHASE					
12	Monday	Off	Off	Off	Off
	Tuesday	Yes	10 min.	Off	Off
	Wednesday	Off	Off	Off	Off
	Thursday	Yes	Off	Off	Off
	Friday	Optional: Choice of one—swim 10 min/bike 20 min/run 15 min			
	Saturday	Off	Off	Off	Off
	Sunday	Off	Off	Off	15 min
11	Monday	Off	Off	Off	Off
	Tuesday	Yes	10 min	Off	Off
	Wednesday	Off	Off	Off	Off
	Thursday	Yes	Off	Off	Off
	Friday	Optional: Choice of one—swim 10 min/bike 20 min/run 15 min.			
	Saturday	Off	Off	30 min	Off
	Sunday	Off	Off	Off	15 min
10	Monday	Off	Off	Off	Off
	Tuesday	Yes	15 min	Off	Off
	Wednesday	Off	Off	Off	Off
	Thursday	Yes	Off	Off	Off
	Friday	Optional: Choice of one—swim 15 min/bike 30 min/run 15 min			
	Saturday	Off	Off	40 min	Off
	Sunday	Off	Off	Off	20 min
9	Monday	Off	Off	Off	Off
	Tuesday	Yes	10 min	Off	Off
	Wednesday	Off	Off	Off	Off
	Thursday	Yes	Off	Off	Off
	Friday	Off	Off	Off	Off
	Saturday	Off	Off	30 min	Off
	Sunday	Off	Off	Off	15 min

Week	Day	Weights	Swim	Bike	Run
BUILD PHASE					
8	Monday	Off	Off	Off	Off
	Tuesday	Yes	15 min	Off	Off
	Wednesday	Off	Off	Off	Off
	Thursday	Yes	Off	Off	Off
	Friday	Optional: Choice of one—swim 15 min/bike 30 min/run 15 min.			
	Saturday	Off	Off	40 min then	5 min
	Sunday	Off	Off	Off	20 min
7	Monday	Off	Off	Off	Off
	Tuesday	Yes	15 min	Off	Off
	Wednesday	Off	Off	Off	Off
	Thursday	Yes	Off	Off	Off
	Friday	Optional: Choice of one—swim 15 min/bike 30 min/run 20 min			
	Saturday	Off	Off	40 min then	5 min
	Sunday	Off	Off	Off	25 min
6	Monday	Off	Off	Off	Off
	Tuesday	Yes	10 min	Off	Off
	Wednesday	Off	Off	Off	Off
	Thursday	Yes	Off	Off	Off
	Friday	Off	Off	Off	Off
	Saturday	Off	Off	30 min	Off
	Sunday	Off	Off	Off	15 min
PEAK PHASE					
5	Monday	Off	Off	Off	Off
	Tuesday	Yes	20 min	Off	Off
	Wednesday	Off	Off	Off	Off
	Thursday	Yes	Off	Off	Off
	Friday	Optional: Choice of one—swim 20 min/bike 30 min/run 20 min			
	Saturday	Off	Off	45 min then	10 min
	Sunday	Off	Off	Off	25 min

Week	Day	Weights	Swim	Bike	Run
PEAK PHASE (continued)					
4	Monday	Off	Off	Off	Off
	Tuesday	Yes	20 min	Off	Off
	Wednesday	Off	Off	Off	Off
	Thursday	Yes	Off	Off	Off
	Friday	Optional: Choice of one—swim 20 min/bike 30 min/run 20 min			
	Saturday	Off	Off	50 min then	10 min
	Sunday	Off	Off	Off	30 min
3	Monday	Off	Off	Off	Off
	Tuesday	Yes	20 min	Off	Off
	Wednesday	Off	Off	Off	Off
	Thursday	Yes	Off	Off	Off
	Friday	Optional: Choice of one—swim 15 min/bike 30 min/run 20 min			
	Saturday	Off	Off	60 min	Off
	Sunday	Off	Off	Off	30 min
TAPER PHASE					
2	Monday	Off	Off	Off	Off
	Tuesday	Off	15 min	Off	Off
	Wednesday	Off	Off	Off	Off
	Thursday	Off	Off	Off	Off
	Friday	Off	Off	Off	Off
	Saturday	Off	Off	40 min then	10 min
	Sunday	Off	Off	Off	20 min
1	Monday	Off	Off	Off	Off
	Tuesday	Off	10 min	Off	Off
	Wednesday	Off	Off	20 min	Off
	Thursday	Off	Off	Off	Off
	Friday	Off	Off	Off	Off
	Saturday	Off	Off	10 min then	5 min
	Sunday	RACE!			

Sprint Distance Program—Performance

Week	Day	Weights	Swim	Bike	Run
BASE PHASE					
12	Monday	Off	Off	Off	Off
	Tuesday	Off	Off	Off	20 min
	Wednesday	Yes	20 min	Off	Off
	Thursday	Off	Off	30 min	Off
	Friday	Yes	20 min	Off	Off
	Saturday	Off	Off	30 min then	5 min
	Sunday	Off	Off	Off	20 min
11	Monday	Off	Off	Off	Off
	Tuesday	Off	Off	Off	20 min
	Wednesday	Yes	20 min	Off	Off
	Thursday	Off	Off	30 min	Off
	Friday	Yes	20 min	Off	Off
	Saturday	Off	Off	30 min then	5 min
	Sunday	Off	Off	Off	20 min
10	Monday	Off	Off	Off	Off
	Tuesday	Off	Off	Off	25 min
	Wednesday	Yes	20 min	Off	Off
	Thursday	Off	Off	40 min	Off
	Friday	Yes	20 min	Off	Off
	Saturday	Off	Off	40 min then	10 min
	Sunday	Off	Off	Off	30 min
9	Monday	Off	Off	Off	Off
	Tuesday	Off	Off	Off	20 min
	Wednesday	Yes	15 min	Off	Off
	Thursday	Off	Off	30 min	Off
	Friday	Yes	15 min	Off	Off
	Saturday	Off	Off	30 min then	5 min
	Sunday	Off	Off	Off	20 min

Week	Day	Weights	Swim	Bike	Run
BUILD PHASE					
8	Monday	Off	Off	Off	Off
	Tuesday	Off	Off	Off	25 min w/5 min RP
	Wednesday	Yes	20 min	Off	Off
	Thursday	Off	Off	30 min w/5 min RP	Off
	Friday	Yes	20 min	Off	Off
	Saturday	Off	Off	45 min w/15 min RP then	10 min
	Sunday	Off	Off	Off	30 min
7	Monday	Off	Off	Off	Off
	Tuesday	Off	Off	Off	25 min w/7 min RP
	Wednesday	Yes	20 min	Off	Off
	Thursday	Off	Off	30 min w/10 min RP	Off
	Friday	Yes	20 min	Off	Off
	Saturday	Off	Off	45 min w/20 min RP then	10 min
	Sunday	Off	Off	Off	20 min
6	Monday	Off	Off	Off	Off
	Tuesday	Off	Off	Off	20 min
	Wednesday	Yes	15 min	Off	Off
	Thursday	Off	Off	30 min	Off
	Friday	Yes	15 min	Off	Off
	Saturday	Off	Off	30 min then	10 min
	Sunday	Off	Off	Off	20 min

Week	Day	Weights	Swim	Bike	Run
PEAK PHASE					
5	Monday	Off	Off	Off	Off
	Tuesday	Off	Off	Off	25 min w/3 min HE
	Wednesday	Yes	20 min	Off	Off
	Thursday	Off	Off	40 min w/5 min HE	Off
	Friday	Yes	20 min	Off	Off
	Saturday	Off	Off	55 min w/10 min JARP then	10 min RP
	Sunday	Off	Off	Off	30 min
4	Monday	Off	Off	Off	Off
	Tuesday	Off	Off	Off	25 min w/2x3 min HE @ 1 min rest
	Wednesday	Yes	20 min	Off	Off
	Thursday	Off	Off	40 min w/2x5 min HE @ 2 min rest	Off
	Friday	Yes	20 min	Off	Off
	Saturday	Off	Off	55 min w/15 min JARP then	10 min RP
	Sunday	Off	Off	Off	30 min
3	Monday	Off	Off	Off	Off
	Tuesday	Off	Off	Off	25 min w/3x3 min HE @ 1 min rest
	Wednesday	Yes	20 min	Off	Off
	Thursday	Off	Off	40 min w/3x5 min HE @ 2 min rest	Off
	Friday	Yes	20 min	Off	Off
	Saturday	Off	Off	55 min w/20 min JARP then	10 min RP
	Sunday	Off	Off	Off	30 min

Week	Day	Weights	Swim	Bike	Run
TAPER PHASE					
2	Monday	Off	Off	Off	Off
	Tuesday	Off	Off	Off	20 min w/3x1 min HE @ 30 sec rest
	Wednesday	Off	15 min	Off	Off
	Thursday	Off	Off	30 min w/5 min HE	Off
	Friday	Off	20 min	Off	Off
	Saturday	Off	Off	30 min w/10 min JARP then	5 min JARP
	Sunday	Off	Off	Off	20 min
1—Saturday Race	Monday	Off	Off	Off	Off
	Tuesday	Off	Off	Off	15 min w/2 min @ HE
	Wednesday	Off	10 min	20 min w/3x1 min HE @ 30 sec rest	Off
	Thursday	Off	Off	Off	Off
	Friday	Off	20 min	10 min then	5 min
	Saturday	RACE!			
	Sunday				
1—Sunday Race	Monday	Off	Off	Off	Off
	Tuesday	Off	Off	Off	15 min w/2 min @ HE
	Wednesday	Off	Off	20 min w/3x1 min HE @ 30 sec rest	Off
	Thursday	Off	10 min	Off	Off
	Friday	Off	Off	Off	Off
	Saturday	Off	Off	10 min then	5 min
	Sunday	RACE!			

Olympic Distance Program

Olympic Distance Program—Finish

Week	Day	Weights	Swim	Bike	Run
BASE PHASE					
12	Monday	Off	Off	Off	Off
	Tuesday	Off	Off	Off	15 min
	Wednesday	Yes	10 min	Off	Off
	Thursday	Off	Off	30 min	Off
	Friday	Yes	10 min	Off	Off
	Saturday	Off	Off	30 min then	5 min
	Sunday	Off	Off	Off	20 min
11	Monday	Off	Off	Off	Off
	Tuesday	Off	Off	Off	15 min
	Wednesday	Yes	10 min	Off	Off
	Thursday	Off	Off	30 min	Off
	Friday	Yes	10 min	Off	Off
	Saturday	Off	Off	30 min then	5 min
	Sunday	Off	Off	Off	20 min
10	Monday	Off	Off	Off	Off
	Tuesday	Off	Off	Off	15 min
	Wednesday	Yes	15 min	Off	Off
	Thursday	Off	Off	30 min	Off
	Friday	Yes	15 min	Off	Off
	Saturday	Off	Off	40 min then	5 min
	Sunday	Off	Off	Off	25 min
9	Monday	Off	Off	Off	Off
	Tuesday	Off	Off	Off	15 min
	Wednesday	Yes	10 min	Off	Off
	Thursday	Off	Off	30 min	Off
	Friday	Yes	10 min	Off	Off
	Saturday	Off	Off	30 min then	5 min
	Sunday	Off	Off	Off	20 min

Week	Day	Weights	Swim	Bike	Run
BUILD PHASE					
8	Monday	Off	Off	Off	Off
	Tuesday	Off	Off	Off	20 min
	Wednesday	Yes	20 min	Off	Off
	Thursday	Off	Off	40 min	Off
	Friday	Yes	20 min	Off	Off
	Saturday	Off	Off	50 min then	5 min
	Sunday	Off	Off	Off	30 min
7	Monday	Off	Off	Off	Off
	Tuesday	Off	Off	Off	20 min
	Wednesday	Yes	25 min	Off	Off
	Thursday	Off	Off	40 min	Off
	Friday	Yes	25 min	Off	Off
	Saturday	Off	Off	60 min then	5 min
	Sunday	Off	Off	Off	35 min
6	Monday	Off	Off	Off	Off
	Tuesday	Off	Off	Off	15 min
	Wednesday	Yes	20 min	Off	Off
	Thursday	Off	Off	30 min	Off
	Friday	Yes	20 min	Off	Off
	Saturday	Off	Off	45 min then	5 min
	Sunday	Off	Off	Off	25 min

Week	Day	Weights	Swim	Bike	Run
PEAK PHASE					
5	Monday	Off	Off	Off	Off
	Tuesday	Off	Off	Off	25 min
	Wednesday	Yes	30 min	Off	Off
	Thursday	Off	Off	45 min	Off
	Friday	Yes	30 min	Off	Off
	Saturday	Off	Off	70 min then	10 min
	Sunday	Off	Off	Off	45 min
4	Monday	Off	Off	Off	Off
	Tuesday	Off	Off	Off	30 min
	Wednesday	Yes	30 min	Off	Off
	Thursday	Off	Off	45 min	Off
	Friday	Yes	30 min	Off	Off
	Saturday	Off	Off	80 min then	10 min
	Sunday	Off	Off	Off	50 min
3	Monday	Off	Off	Off	Off
	Tuesday	Off	Off	Off	30 min
	Wednesday	Yes	30 min	Off	Off
	Thursday	Off	Off	45 min	Off
	Friday	Yes	30 min	Off	Off
	Saturday	Off	Off	80 min then	10 min
	Sunday	Off	Off	Off	55 min

Week	Day	Weights	Swim	Bike	Run
TAPER PHASE					
2	Monday	Off	Off	Off	Off
	Tuesday	Off	Off	Off	20 min
	Wednesday	Off	20 min	Off	Off
	Thursday	Off	Off	30 min	Off
	Friday	Off	20 min	Off	Off
	Saturday	Off	Off	50 min then	10 min
	Sunday	Off	Off	Off	30 min
1—Saturday Race	Monday	Off	Off	Off	Off
	Tuesday	Off	10 min	Off	20 min
	Wednesday	Off	Off	20 min	Off
	Thursday	Off	Off	Off	Off
	Friday	Off	Off	15 min	5 min
	Saturday	RACE!			
	Sunday				
1—Sunday Race	Monday	Off	Off	Off	Off
	Tuesday	Off	Off	Off	20 min
	Wednesday	Off	10 min	Off	Off
	Thursday	Off	Off	20 min	Off
	Friday	Off	Off	Off	Off
	Saturday	Off	Off	15 min	5 min
	Sunday	RACE!			

Olympic Distance Program—Performance

Week	Day	Weights	Swim	Bike	Run
BASE PHASE					
12	Monday	Off	Off	Off	Off
	Tuesday	Off	Off	Off	30 min
	Wednesday	Yes	30 min	Off	Off
	Thursday	Off	Off	30 min	Off
	Friday	Yes	30 min	Off	Off
	Saturday	Off	Off	45 min then	10 min
	Sunday	Off	Off	Off	40 min
11	Monday	Off	Off	Off	Off
	Tuesday	Off	Off	Off	30 min
	Wednesday	Yes	30 min	Off	Off
	Thursday	Off	Off	30 min	Off
	Friday	Yes	30 min	Off	Off
	Saturday	Off	Off	45 min then	10 min
	Sunday	Off	Off	Off	40 min
10	Monday	Off	Off	Off	Off
	Tuesday	Off	Off	Off	30 min
	Wednesday	Yes	30 min	Off	Off
	Thursday	Off	Off	45 min	Off
	Friday	Yes	30 min	Off	Off
	Saturday	Off	Off	55 min then	10 min
	Sunday	Off	Off	Off	50 min
9	Monday	Off	Off	Off	Off
	Tuesday	Off	Off	Off	30 min
	Wednesday	Yes	30 min	Off	Off
	Thursday	Off	Off	30 min	Off
	Friday	Yes	30 min	Off	Off
	Saturday	Off	Off	45 min then	10 min
	Sunday	Off	Off	Off	40 min

Week	Day	Weights	Swim	Bike	Run
BUILD PHASE					
8	Monday	Off	Off	Off	Off
	Tuesday	Off	Off	Off	30 min w/15 min RP
	Wednesday	Yes	30 min	Off	Off
	Thursday	Off	Off	45 min w/15 min RP	Off
	Friday	Yes	30 min	Off	Off
	Saturday	Off	Off	60 min w/ 25 min RP then	10 min RP
	Sunday	Off	Off	Off	50 min
7	Monday	Off	Off	Off	Off
	Tuesday	Off	Off	Off	40 min w/20 min RP
	Wednesday	Yes	30 min	Off	Off
	Thursday	Off	Off	45 min w/20 min RP	Off
	Friday	Yes	30 min	Off	Off
	Saturday	Off	Off	75 min w/35 min RP then	10 min RP
	Sunday	Off	Off	Off	60 min
6	Monday	Off	Off	Off	Off
	Tuesday	Off	Off	Off	30 min
	Wednesday	Yes	30 min	Off	Off
	Thursday	Off	Off	45 min	Off
	Friday	Yes	30 min	Off	Off
	Saturday	Off	Off	60 min then	10 min
	Sunday	Off	Off	Off	45 min

Week	Day	Weights	Swim	Bike	Run
PEAK PHASE					
5	Monday	Off	Off	Off	Off
	Tuesday	Off	Off	Off	40 min w/4 min HE
	Wednesday	Yes	30 min	Off	Off
	Thursday	Off	Off	60 min w/5 min HE	Off
	Friday	Yes	30 min	Off	Off
	Saturday	Off	Off	90 min w/20 min JARP then	15 min JARP
	Sunday	Off	Off	Off	60 min
4	Monday	Off	Off	Off	Off
	Tuesday	Off	Off	Off	40 min w/2x4 min HE @ 2 min rest
	Wednesday	Yes	30 min	Off	Off
	Thursday	Off	Off	60 min w/2x5 min HE @ 2 min rest	Off
	Friday	Yes	30 min	Off	Off
	Saturday	Off	Off	90 min w/25 min JARP then	15 min JARP
	Sunday	Off	Off	Off	60 min
3	Monday	Off	Off	Off	Off
	Tuesday	Off	Off	Off	40 min w/3x4 min HE @ 2 min rest
	Wednesday	Yes	30 min	Off	Off
	Thursday	Off	Off	60 min w/3x5 min HE @ 2 min rest	Off
	Friday	Yes	30 min	Off	Off
	Saturday	Off	Off	90 min w/30 min JARP then	15 min JARP
	Sunday	Off	Off	Off	60 min

Week	Day	Weights	Swim	Bike	Run
TAPER PHASE					
2	Monday	Off	Off	Off	Off
	Tuesday	Off	Off	Off	30 min w/3x2 min HE @ 1 min rest
	Wednesday	Off	30 min	Off	Off
	Thursday	Off	Off	45 min w/5 min HE	Off
	Friday	Off	30 min	Off	Off
	Saturday	Off	Off	60 min w/10 min JARP then	15 min JARP
	Sunday	Off	Off	Off	45 min
1—Saturday Race	Monday	Off	Off	Off	Off
	Tuesday	Off	Off	Off	20 min w/3 min HE @ 30 sec rest
	Wednesday	Off	15 min	30 min w/3x1 min HE @ 30 sec rest	Off
	Thursday	Off	Off	Off	Off
	Friday	Off	Off	15 min then	10 min
	Saturday	RACE!			
	Sunday				
1—Sunday Race	Monday	Off	Off	Off	Off
	Tuesday	Off	Off	Off	20 min w/3 min HE @ 30 sec rest
	Wednesday	Off	Off	30 min w/3x1 min HE @ 30 sec rest	Off
	Thursday	Off	15 min	Off	Off
	Friday	Off	Off	Off	Off
	Saturday	Off	Off	15 min then	10 min
	Sunday	RACE!			

Half-Ironman Distance Program

Half-Ironman Distance Program—Finish

Week	Day	Weights	Swim	Bike	Run
BASE PHASE					
12	Monday	Off	Off	Off	Off
	Tuesday	Off	Off	Off	30 min
	Wednesday	Yes	20 min	Off	Off
	Thursday	Off	Off	45 min	Off
	Friday	Yes	20 min	Off	Off
	Saturday	Off	Off	60 min then	15 min
	Sunday	Off	Off	Off	45 min
11	Monday	Off	Off	Off	Off
	Tuesday	Off	Off	Off	30 min
	Wednesday	Yes	20 min	Off	Off
	Thursday	Off	Off	45 min	Off
	Friday	Yes	20 min	Off	Off
	Saturday	Off	Off	60 min then	15 min
	Sunday	Off	Off	Off	45 min
10	Monday	Off	Off	Off	Off
	Tuesday	Off	Off	Off	30 min
	Wednesday	Yes	25 min	Off	Off
	Thursday	Off	Off	60 min	Off
	Friday	Yes	25 min	Off	Off
	Saturday	Off	Off	75 min then	15 min
	Sunday	Off	Off	Off	55 min
9	Monday	Off	Off	Off	Off
	Tuesday	Off	Off	Off	30 min
	Wednesday	Yes	20 min	Off	Off
	Thursday	Off	Off	45 min	Off
	Friday	Yes	20 min	Off	Off
	Saturday	Off	Off	60 min then	15 min
	Sunday	Off	Off	Off	45 min

Week	Day	Weights	Swim	Bike	Run
BUILD PHASE					
8	Monday	Off	Off	Off	Off
	Tuesday	Off	Off	Off	30 min
	Wednesday	Yes	30 min	Off	Off
	Thursday	Off	Off	60 min	Off
	Friday	Yes	30 min	Off	Off
	Saturday	Off	Off	75 min then	15 min
	Sunday	Off	Off	Off	60 min
7	Monday	Off	Off	Off	Off
	Tuesday	Off	Off	Off	40 min
	Wednesday	Yes	30 min	Off	Off
	Thursday	Off	Off	60 min	Off
	Friday	Yes	30 min	Off	Off
	Saturday	Off	Off	2 hr then	15 min
	Sunday	Off	Off	Off	75 min
6	Monday	Off	Off	Off	Off
	Tuesday	Off	Off	Off	25 min
	Wednesday	Yes	20 min	Off	Off
	Thursday	Off	Off	45 min	Off
	Friday	Yes	20 min	Off	Off
	Saturday	Off	Off	60 min then	15 min
	Sunday	Off	Off	Off	45 min

Week	Day	Weights	Swim	Bike	Run
PEAK PHASE					
5	Monday	Off	Off	Off	Off
	Tuesday	Off	Off	Off	45 min
	Wednesday	Yes	40 min	Off	Off
	Thursday	Off	Off	60 min	Off
	Friday	Yes	40 min	Off	Off
	Saturday	Off	Off	2.25 hr then	30 min
	Sunday	Off	Off	Off	90 min
4	Monday	Off	Off	Off	Off
	Tuesday	Off	Off	Off	45 min
	Wednesday	Yes	40 min	Off	Off
	Thursday	Off	Off	60 min	Off
	Friday	Yes	40 min	Off	Off
	Saturday	Off	Off	2.5 hr then	30 min
	Sunday	Off	Off	Off	105 min
3	Monday	Off	Off	Off	Off
	Tuesday	Off	Off	Off	45 min
	Wednesday	Yes	40 min	Off	Off
	Thursday	Off	Off	60 min	Off
	Friday	Yes	40 min	Off	Off
	Saturday	Off	Off	3 hr then	30 min
	Sunday	Off	Off	Off	2 hr

Week	Day	Weights	Swim	Bike	Run
TAPER PHASE					
2	Monday	Off	Off	Off	Off
	Tuesday	Off	Off	Off	30 min
	Wednesday	Off	30 min	Off	Off
	Thursday	Off	Off	45 min	Off
	Friday	Off	30 min	Off	Off
	Saturday	Off	Off	90 min then	30 min
	Sunday	Off	Off	Off	60 min
1—Saturday Race	Monday	Off	Off	Off	Off
	Tuesday	Off	Off	30 min	Off
	Wednesday	Off	20 min	Off	20 min
	Thursday	Off	Off	Off	Off
	Friday	Off	Off	20 min	10 min
	Saturday	RACE!			
	Sunday				
1—Sunday Race	Monday	Off	Off	Off	Off
	Tuesday	Off	Off	Off	20 min
	Wednesday	Off	Off	30 min	Off
	Thursday	Off	20 min	Off	Off
	Friday	Off	Off	Off	Off
	Saturday	Off	Off	20 min	10 min
	Sunday	RACE!			

Half-Ironman Distance Program—Performance

Week	Day	Weights	Swim	Bike	Run
BASE PHASE					
12	Monday	Off	Off	Off	Off
	Tuesday	Off	30 min	Off	30 min
	Wednesday	Yes	Off	60 min	Off
	Thursday	Off	Off	45 min then	15 min
	Friday	Yes	30 min	Off	Off
	Saturday	Off	Off	60 min then	30 min
	Sunday	Off	Off	Off	45 min
11	Monday	Off	Off	Off	Off
	Tuesday	Off	30 min	Off	30 min
	Wednesday	Yes	Off	60 min	Off
	Thursday	Off	Off	45 min then	15 min
	Friday	Yes	30 min	Off	Off
	Saturday	Off	Off	60 min then	30 min
	Sunday	Off	Off	Off	45 min
10	Monday	Off	Off	Off	Off
	Tuesday	Off	45 min	Off	40 min
	Wednesday	Yes	Off	60 min	Off
	Thursday	Off	Off	60 min then	15 min
	Friday	Yes	45 min	Off	Off
	Saturday	Off	Off	90 min then	30 min
	Sunday	Off	Off	Off	60 min
9	Monday	Off	Off	Off	Off
	Tuesday	Off	30 min	Off	30 min
	Wednesday	Yes	Off	60 min	Off
	Thursday	Off	Off	45 min then	15 min
	Friday	Yes	30 min	Off	Off
	Saturday	Off	Off	60 min then	30 min
	Sunday	Off	Off	Off	45 min

Week	Day	Weights	Swim	Bike	Run
BUILD PHASE					
8	Monday	Off	Off	Off	Off
	Tuesday	Off	45 min	Off	4x800s @ 2 min rest
	Wednesday	Yes	Off	60 min w/20 min RP	Off
	Thursday	Off	Off	60 min w/20 min RP then	15 min
	Friday	Yes	45 min	Off	Off
	Saturday	Off	Off	90 min w/30 min RP then	30 min
	Sunday	Off	Off	Off	60 min
7	Monday	Off	Off	Off	Off
	Tuesday	Off	45 min	Off	6x800s @ 2 min rest
	Wednesday	Yes	Off	60 min w/30 min RP	Off
	Thursday	Off	Off	60 min w/30 min RP then	15 min
	Friday	Yes	45 min	Off	Off
	Saturday	Off	Off	2 hr w/45 min RP then	30 min
	Sunday	Off	Off	Off	75 min
6	Monday	Off	Off	Off	Off
	Tuesday	Off	30 min	Off	40 min
	Wednesday	Yes	Off	45 min	Off
	Thursday	Off	Off	45 min then	15 min
	Friday	Yes	45 min	Off	Off
	Saturday	Off	Off	60 min then	30 min
	Sunday	Off	Off	Off	45 min

Week	Day	Weights	Swim	Bike	Run
PEAK PHASE					
5	Monday	Off	Off	Off	Off
	Tuesday	Off	45 min	Off	6x400s @ 30 sec rest
	Wednesday	Yes	Off	60 min w/5 min HE	Off
	Thursday	Off	Off	60 min w/10 min JARP then	15 min JARP
	Friday	Yes	45 min	Off	Off
	Saturday	Off	Off	2.5 hr w/60 min RP then	30 min RP
	Sunday	Off	Off	Off	90 min
4	Monday	Off	Off	Off	Off
	Tuesday	Off	45 min	Off	7x400s @ 30 sec rest
	Wednesday	Yes	Off	60 min w/2x5 min HE @ 2 min rest	Off
	Thursday	Off	Off	60 min w/15 min JARP then	15 min JARP
	Friday	Yes	45 min	Off	Off
	Saturday	Off	Off	3 hr w/90 min RP then	30 min RP
	Sunday	Off	Off	Off	105 min
3	Monday	Off	Off	Off	Off
	Tuesday	Off	45 min	Off	8x400s @ 30 sec rest
	Wednesday	Yes	Off	60 min w/3x5 min HE @ 2 min rest	Off
	Thursday	Off	Off	60 min w/20 min JARP then	15 min JARP
	Friday	Yes	45 min	Off	Off
	Saturday	Off	Off	3 hr w/2 hr RP then	45 min RP
	Sunday	Off	Off	Off	2 hr

Week	Day	Weights	Swim	Bike	Run
TAPER PHASE					
2	Monday	Off	Off	Off	Off
	Tuesday	Off	30 min	Off	40 min w/3x2 min HE @ 1 min rest
	Wednesday	Off	Off	45 min w/5 min HE	Off
	Thursday	Off	Off	45 min w/10 min JARP then	15 min RP
	Friday	Off	30 min	Off	Off
	Saturday	Off	Off	90 min w/45 min RP then	30 min RP
	Sunday	Off	Off	Off	60 min
1—Saturday Race	Monday	Off	Off	Off	Off
	Tuesday	Off	20 min	Off	30 min w/3x1 min HE @ 30 sec rest
	Wednesday	Off	Off	30 min w/10 min JARP	Off
	Thursday	Off	Off	Off	Off
	Friday	Off	Off	20 min then	10 min
	Saturday	RACE!			
	Sunday				
1—Sundayday Race	Monday	Off	Off	Off	Off
	Tuesday	Off	Off	Off	30 min w/3x1 min HE @ 30 sec rest
	Wednesday	Off	20 min	Off	Off
	Thursday	Off	Off	30 min w/10 min JARP	Off
	Friday	Off	Off	Off	Off
	Saturday	Off	Off	20 min then	10 min
	Sunday	RACE!			

Ironman Distance Program

Ironman Distance Program—Finish

Week	Day	Weights	Swim	Bike	Run
BASE PHASE					
12	Monday	Off	Off	Off	Off
	Tuesday	Off	Off	Off	30 min
	Wednesday	Yes	30 min	Off	Off
	Thursday	Off	Off	45 min	Off
	Friday	Yes	30 min	Off	Off
	Saturday	Off	Off	60 min then	30 min
	Sunday	Off	Off	Off	45 min
11	Monday	Off	Off	Off	Off
	Tuesday	Off	Off	Off	30 min
	Wednesday	Yes	30 min	Off	Off
	Thursday	Off	Off	45 min	Off
	Friday	Yes	30 min	Off	Off
	Saturday	Off	Off	60 min then	30 min
	Sunday	Off	Off	Off	45 min
10	Monday	Off	Off	Off	Off
	Tuesday	Off	Off	Off	40 min
	Wednesday	Yes	40 min	Off	Off
	Thursday	Off	Off	60 min	Off
	Friday	Yes	40 min	Off	Off
	Saturday	Off	Off	90 min then	30 min
	Sunday	Off	Off	Off	60 min
9	Monday	Off	Off	Off	Off
	Tuesday	Off	Off	Off	30 min
	Wednesday	Yes	30 min	Off	Off
	Thursday	Off	Off	45 min	Off
	Friday	Yes	30 min	Off	Off
	Saturday	Off	Off	60 min then	30 min
	Sunday	Off	Off	Off	45 min

Week	Day	Weights	Swim	Bike	Run
BUILD PHASE					
8	Monday	Off	Off	Off	Off
	Tuesday	Off	Off	Off	45 min
	Wednesday	Yes	50 min	Off	Off
	Thursday	Off	Off	90 min	Off
	Friday	Yes	50 min	Off	Off
	Saturday	Off	Off	2 hr then	45 min
	Sunday	Off	Off	Off	90 min
7	Monday	Off	Off	Off	Off
	Tuesday	Off	Off	Off	45 min
	Wednesday	Yes	50 min	Off	Off
	Thursday	Off	Off	90 min	Off
	Friday	Yes	50 min	Off	Off
	Saturday	Off	Off	3 hr then	45 min
	Sunday	Off	Off	Off	2 hr
6	Monday	Off	Off	Off	Off
	Tuesday	Off	Off	Off	30 min
	Wednesday	Yes	30 min	Off	Off
	Thursday	Off	Off	60 min	Off
	Friday	Yes	30 min	Off	Off
	Saturday	Off	Off	2 hr then	30 min
	Sunday	Off	Off	Off	60 min

Week	Day	Weights	Swim	Bike	Run
PEAK PHASE					
5	Monday	Off	Off	Off	Off
	Tuesday	Off	Off	Off	60 min
	Wednesday	Yes	60 min	Off	Off
	Thursday	Off	Off	2 hr	Off
	Friday	Yes	60 min	Off	Off
	Saturday	Off	Off	4 hr then	60 min
	Sunday	Off	Off	Off	2 hr
4	Monday	Off	Off	Off	Off
	Tuesday	Off	Off	Off	60 min
	Wednesday	Yes	60 min	Off	Off
	Thursday	Off	Off	2 hr	Off
	Friday	Yes	60 min	Off	Off
	Saturday	Off	Off	5 hr then	60 min
	Sunday	Off	Off	Off	2.5 hr
3	Monday	Off	Off	Off	Off
	Tuesday	Off	Off	Off	60 min
	Wednesday	Yes	60 min	Off	Off
	Thursday	Off	Off	2 hr	Off
	Friday	Yes	60 min	Off	Off
	Saturday	Off	Off	6 hr then	60 min
	Sunday	Off	Off	Off	3 hr

Week	Day	Weights	Swim	Bike	Run
TAPER PHASE					
2	Monday	Off	Off	Off	Off
	Tuesday	Off	Off	Off	40 min
	Wednesday	Yes	45 min	Off	Off
	Thursday	Off	Off	90 min	Off
	Friday	Yes	45 min	Off	Off
	Saturday	Off	Off	3 hr then	30 min
	Sunday	Off	Off	Off	90 min
1—Saturday Race	Monday	Off	Off	Off	Off
	Tuesday	Off	Off	30 min	Off
	Wednesday	Off	20 min	Off	20 min
	Thursday	Off	Off	Off	Off
	Friday	Off	Off	20 min then	10 min
	Saturday	RACE!			
	Sunday				
1—Sunday Race	Monday	Off	Off	Off	Off
	Tuesday	Off	Off	Off	20 min
	Wednesday	Off	Off	30 min	Off
	Thursday	Off	20 min	Off	Off
	Friday	Off	Off	Off	Off
	Saturday	Off	Off	20 min then	10 min
	Sunday	RACE!			

Ironman Distance Program—Performance

Week	Day	Weights	Swim	Bike	Run
BASE PHASE					
12	Monday	Off	Off	Off	Off
	Tuesday	Off	45 min	Off	30 min
	Wednesday	Yes	Off	60 min	Off
	Thursday	Off	Off	60 min then	30 min
	Friday	Yes	45 min	Off	40 min
	Saturday	Off	Off	2 hr then	30 min
	Sunday	Off	Off	Off	60 min
11	Monday	Off	Off	Off	Off
	Tuesday	Off	45 min	Off	30 min
	Wednesday	Yes	Off	60 min	Off
	Thursday	Off	Off	60 min then	30 min
	Friday	Yes	45 min	Off	40 min
	Saturday	Off	Off	2 hr then	30 min
	Sunday	Off	Off	Off	60 min
10	Monday	Off	Off	Off	Off
	Tuesday	Off	60 min	Off	40 min
	Wednesday	Yes	Off	90 min	Off
	Thursday	Off	Off	90 min then	30 min
	Friday	Yes	60 min	Off	40 min
	Saturday	Off	Off	3 hr then	30 min
	Sunday	Off	Off	Off	90 min
9	Monday	Off	Off	Off	Off
	Tuesday	Off	45 min	Off	30 min
	Wednesday	Yes	Off	60 min	Off
	Thursday	Off	Off	60 min then	30 min
	Friday	Yes	45 min	Off	40 min
	Saturday	Off	Off	2 hr then	30 min
	Sunday	Off	Off	Off	60 min

Week	Day	Weights	Swim	Bike	Run	
BUILD PHASE						
8	Monday	Off	Off	Off	Off	Off
	Tuesday	Off	60 min	Off	4x1 mi @ 2 min rest	
	Wednesday	Yes	Off	90 min w/30 min RP	Off	
	Thursday	Off	Off	90 min w/30 min RP then	30 min	
	Friday	Yes	60 min	Off	50 min w/10 min JARP	
	Saturday	Off	Off	4 hr w/60 min RP then	45 min	
	Sunday	Off	Off	Off	90 min	
7	Monday	Off	Off	Off	Off	
	Tuesday	Off	60 min	Off	5x1 mi @ 2 min rest	
	Wednesday	Yes	Off	2 hr w/45 min @ RP	Off	
	Thursday	Off	Off	2 hr w/45 min @ RP then	30 min	
	Friday	Yes	60 min	Off	60 min w/15 min JARP	
	Saturday	Off	Off	5 hr w/2 hr RP then	45 min	
	Sunday	Off	Off	Off	2 hr	
6	Monday	Off	Off	Off	Off	
	Tuesday	Off	60 min	Off	30 min	
	Wednesday	Yes	Off	60 min	Off	
	Thursday	Off	Off	60 min then	30 min	
	Friday	Yes	60 min	Off	30 min	
	Saturday	Off	Off	3 hr then	30 min	
	Sunday	Off	Off	Off	60 min	

Week	Day	Weights	Swim	Bike	Run
PEAK PHASE					
5	Monday	Off	Off	Off	Off
	Tuesday	Off	60 min	Off	6x1 mi @ 2 min rest
	Wednesday	Yes	Off	2 hr w/10 min HE	Off
	Thursday	Off	Off	2 hr w/20 min JARP then	30 min JARP
	Friday	Yes	60 min	Off	60 min w/20 min JARP
	Saturday	Off	Off	5 hr w/3 hr RP then	60 min
	Sunday	Off	Off	Off	2.25 hr
4	Monday	Off	Off	Off	Off
	Tuesday	Off	60 min	Off	6x1 mi @ 2 min rest
	Wednesday	Yes	Off	2 hr w/2x10 min HE @ 5 min rest	Off
	Thursday	Off	Off	2 hr w/30 min JARP then	30 min JARP
	Friday	Yes	60 min	Off	60 min w/25 min JARP
	Saturday	Off	Off	100 miles then	60 min
	Sunday	Off	Off	Off	2.5 hr
3	Monday	Off	Off	Off	Off
	Tuesday	Off	60 min	Off	4x800s @ 1 min rest
	Wednesday	Yes	Off	2 hr w/3x5 min HE @ 2 min rest	Off
	Thursday	Off	Off	2 hr w/30 min JARP then	30 min JARP
	Friday	Yes	60 min	Off	60 min w/30 min JARP
	Saturday	Off	Off	100 miles then	60 min
	Sunday	Off	Off	Off	20 miles

Week	Day	Weights	Swim	Bike	Run
TAPER PHASE					
2	Monday	Off	Off	Off	Off
	Tuesday	Off	45 min	Off	4x400s @ 30 sec rest
	Wednesday	Yes	Off	60 min w/5 min HE	Off
	Thursday	Off	Off	60 min w/20 min JARP then	30 min JARP
	Friday	Yes	45 min	Off	Off
	Saturday	Off	Off	3 hr w/2 hr RP then	30 min JARP
	Sunday	Off	Off	Off	90 min
1—Saturday Race	Monday	Off	Off	Off	Off
	Tuesday	Off	30 min	Off	30 min
	Wednesday	Off	Off	60 min	Off
	Thursday	Off	Off	Off	Off
	Friday	Off	Off	20 min then	10 min
	Saturday	RACE!			
	Sunday				
1—Sunday Race	Monday	Off	Off	Off	Off
	Tuesday	Off	Off	Off	30 min
	Wednesday	Off	30 min	Off	Off
	Thursday	Off	Off	60 min	Off
	Friday	Off	Off	Off	Off
	Saturday	Off	Off	20 min then	10 min
	Sunday	RACE!			

Can I switch days if I have to—for example, do my Sunday workout on Saturday and my Saturday workout on Sunday?

Yes. Family, work, and travel will inevitably come up and force you to make some adaptations. This is unavoidable and you may therefore swap days if you need to. There is a method to the madness in the progression of the workouts, however, so it is best to follow it as closely as possible whenever possible. If you happen to work on Saturdays and have Wednesdays off and want to do your brick workout midweek, then that is when you will do it. Once again, the goal is to be consistent with all areas of your training and not skip the workouts or sports that you don't enjoy as much.

What if I miss a workout? Should I make it up the next day or just skip it?

You will by no means do 100 percent of these workouts—it is virtually impossible, and I, as both a coach and an athlete, realize this. Do not beat yourself up if you miss a workout; it happens. Your key workouts are your weekend brick and your long run. If you miss a workout during the week, then just stick with the schedule and do the next day's session. If you miss a weekend workout, then I would try to make it up as early as possible. In other words, if you are traveling on Saturday and cannot get that workout in, then that becomes your Monday off day. You can then do Saturday's workout on Sunday and Sunday's workout on Monday instead.

Be flexible and be smart. Make sure you are not consistently missing a workout because that is a workout you don't particularly enjoy. Work on your weaknesses until they become your strengths. As my Sports Psychology professor loved to say, "If you want to know what your weaknesses are, just ask your competition."

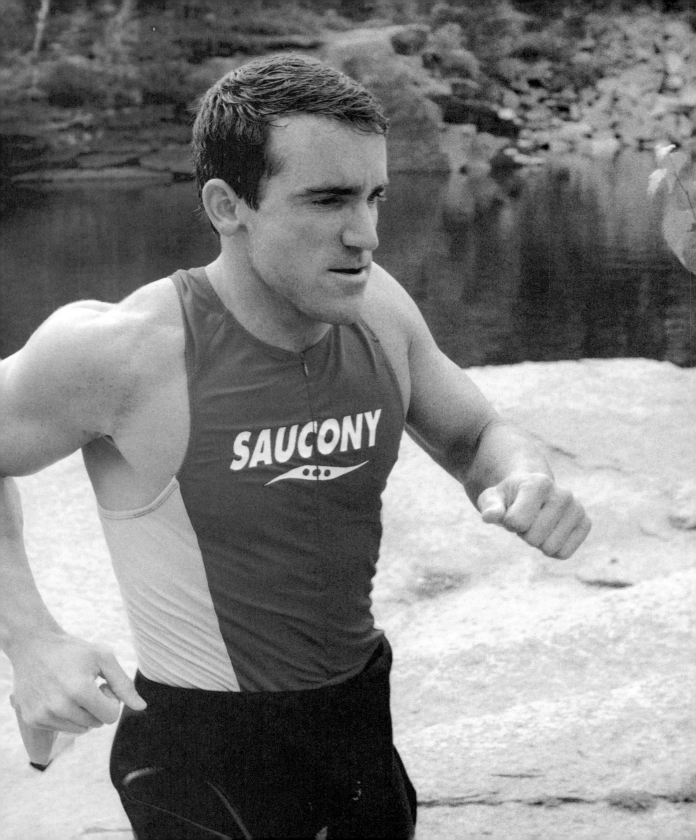

CHAPTER 10
Mental Training

The mental side of sports performance, especially endurance sports, is one of my real passions, and that is why I pursued sport psychology as part of my master's degree. I would argue that, at every Hawaii Ironman, the top pros are at essentially the same level physiologically as the other competitors; however, it is the man and woman who have the best control of their mental game who will inevitably take home the victory. You need to be in control of your mental game as well. Sport psychology is a complex and broad field, and therefore I will condense these concepts down to fit into a framework for you, the 12-Week Triathlete. After all, you will already be swimming, biking, running, lifting weights, and stretching; adding in a complex and time-consuming mental component is not realistic or necessary.

But make no mistake about it, you will want to read through this chapter and apply the principles as best you can. They are simple and will not take up much time. Like everything else in your training, the key to success is consistency. No matter how consistently or hard you train physically, your race can be disastrous if you lose control of your mental game. Conversely, you can impact your race in incredibly positive ways by using mental techniques and training as well.

There is a mental component that you will engage in during your training as well as mental techniques that you will call upon on race day. Relaxation and visualization are the two mental training tools that you will practice before your triathlon that will benefit you enormously during your triathlon. Self-talk is the mental tool that you will use to increase your performance as well as enjoyment on the day of the race.

RELAXATION EXERCISE AND TRAINING

"Arousal," or in layman's terms, how "psyched-up" you are for a race, has two distinct characteristics as it applies to sports performance:

1. It is highly individualistic.
2. There is an Inverted-U Theory between arousal and performance.

It is individualistic in the sense that your optimal state of arousal is not necessarily the same as your competitor's. In other words, you may perform better when you are a little more excited, whereas that same level of excitement might be too high or too low for someone else. One athlete may listen to classical music to bring himself to his optimal state of arousal, whereas another may prefer heavy metal. One may yell out loud to get herself "psyched up," whereas another prefers to be alone and not speak before her race. You need to uncover and find your own personal optimal state of arousal.

The Inverted-U Theory is actually simpler than it sounds. It means that you can be

THE POWER OF THE MIND

Back in the '50s, it was believed that running a sub-four-minute mile was physiologically impossible. Well, as many now know, Roger Bannister was the first person to break this barrier and prove this theory to be incorrect. While the achievement is in itself incredible, what I believe is most noteworthy about this event is what happened soon after Roger Bannister's accomplishment. John Landy, Bannister's main competition at the time, went on to run a sub-four-minute mile just forty-six days later, and many followed soon after. What changed so quickly? Training? A magic supplement? No; suddenly people believed that it could be done, whereas before, they did not. Henry Ford said it best: "Whether you think you can or think you can't, you are right."

either too excited or too relaxed before your event, and both of these states will negatively affect your performance. Yes, you can be too relaxed before a triathlon!

Great coaches know that their athletes all have different optimal levels of arousal. They learn where each particular athlete lies on this Inverted-U and determine what he or she needs to get there.

What you want to do is practice short relaxation exercises during your twelve weeks of training, starting during the first week. Relaxation exercises will not be effective if you try to practice them a week or two out from your triathlon. If you do practice them consistently, you will be able to utilize the technique to calm yourself in the most stressful of conditions.

While the ability to calm yourself may be useful at any time during a triathlon, there are two primary situations in which I believe it is the most useful to the triathlete: the race start and during the swim.

Both of these situations are generally ones in which athletes may experience the most stress. As far as the race start is concerned, I'll never forget standing on the beach before the start of a Half-Ironman and listening to the audible sound of the heart rate monitor on one of the triathletes next to me. We were all standing motionless as "The Star-Spangled Banner" played, yet the incredibly fast beeping of this athlete's monitor signified that his heart rate was approaching anaerobic levels from sheer anxiety alone. Once again, everyone is nervous before a race, and a little nervousness is, indeed, good (remember, you can be too relaxed!), but this level of anxiety most likely had him way above his optimal level of arousal. Having practiced relaxation exercises and using them at that time would have benefited him greatly. Just before a race start, our body generally enters the fight-or-flight mode, and we can really benefit by lowering the effects of this reaction. This is where relaxation exercises come in.

During the actual swim is another situation where I believe calling upon relaxation exercises can be extremely helpful. Now you not only have the stress and adrenaline from the actual race start to contend with, but you also have numerous other potential stressors that come with swimming in a pack, such as the punching and kicking, not to mention the common fear of sharks and other sea life when swimming in the ocean. All of these things can elevate the heart rate and create incredible anxiety, even to the point of panic attacks. Yes, there are usually at least several people who need to be pulled out of the water at most triathlons due to panic attacks. Learning to calm oneself through relaxation exercises can help to prevent these occurrences as well as drastically improve your swim experience and enjoyment.

SIMPLE RELAXATION EXERCISE

Again, this should not take a great deal of time. Three times a week for three to five minutes per session is a great place to begin.

1. Try to find a quiet place.
2. Sit or lie in a comfortable position.
3. Close your eyes.
4. Begin to breathe in deeply through your nose and exhale through your mouth.
5. Visualize a calm scene. It can be anything you choose—a location, a face, an object, anything that brings about an incredibly calm feeling.
6. Focus on the scene while trying to keep all other thoughts from your mind.
7. Pick one word that also has a calming effect on you and begin to hear it repeated over and over as you continue to breathe deeply.
8. Continue this for several minutes or until you significantly lose focus.

That's it. It may seem ridiculous, but if you practice this consistently, you will be able to effectively calm yourself both before and during your race by calling upon this image, this word, or both.

VISUALIZATION EXERCISES

One of my favorite concepts in sport psychology is visualization, also known as imagery or mental practice. Simply put, it is the act of "practicing" in your mind, "visualizing" yourself performing your sport. I would argue that the majority of the top athletes in all sports practice some form of mental training. Like relaxation exercises, visualization exercises should be practiced throughout the course of your training. These sessions do not require a great deal of time either, and can bring about extraordinary results. Research has shown that mental training along with physical training can indeed lead to increased sport performance.

When performing visualization exercises, you will "see" yourself performing on race day. You will visualize yourself performing effortlessly, with perfect form, essentially having the "race of your life." You picture yourself swimming your best, biking your best, and running your best.

Your visualization should not be limited to merely swimming, biking, and running, either. You should visualize yourself arriving at the race, in the transition area, and waiting for the gun to start the race. You should also "see" yourself crossing the finish line, "seeing" the clock reading your time goal if you have set one for yourself.

How to Practice Visualization

There are two ways to visualize: from a first-person or from a third-person perspective. When using a first-person perspective, you are picturing the scene as though through your own eyes; a third-person perspective is similar to your being filmed, seen through the "camera's eye," seeing yourself from the perspective of a camera or spectator. Most people naturally choose one perspective—I recommend trying to practice both types.

1. Begin as you would your relaxation exercises. Find a quite place, get comfortable, close your eyes, and begin breathing deeply.

2. Begin to visualize yourself in a triathlon situation—attending to prerace tasks; swimming, biking, or running; or at the race finish. See yourself confident, strong, and calm, performing flawlessly and with unlimited energy.

3. Try to utilize all of your senses. The more senses you use, the more effective the visualization will be. For example, if you are visualizing yourself running from a first-person perspective, you will "see" the road in front of you, the people you are slowly passing, the spectators lining the sides of the course; you "hear" the sound of yourself breathing comfortably, your feet hitting the road lightly, the crowd cheering you on; you "smell" the Gatorade that you have inevitably spilled on yourself; you "feel" your body running relaxed with low shoulders, smooth arm swing, and soft foot strike; and you "taste" the sweat as it drips into your mouth, mixing with the lingering taste of Gatorade that you have learned to love.

4. Try to practice visualizing several times a week for three to ten minutes per session.

By practicing visualization, you will potentially improve your technique, increase your confidence level, and ultimately improve your race performance.

SELF-TALK

The textbook definition of self-talk is "An effective technique for controlling thoughts and influencing feelings, both of which can influence self-confidence as well as performance." Self-talk is our own internal monologue, the "conversations" we have with ourselves in our minds. They are your thoughts, your affirmations, your personal mantras. Anyone who has participated in a long endurance race has experienced the phenomenon of being all alone on the course and having long conversations with him- or herself, all in his or her head.

Self-talk is an incredible concept, and I believe it to be an essential tool in both sports performance as well as enjoyment. The thoughts we have in our mind play such a crucial role in how our body feels, and we can control this relationship.

To illustrate the incredible mind/body connection, I often use this example during my lectures on the topic of self-talk:

Close your eyes. Imagine that you are in your kitchen. See yourself walk to the refrigerator and open it. You take out a big fat lemon and carry it to the counter. You take a knife out of a drawer and cut the lemon in half, then cut the pieces in half again. See the lemon juice that has spilled onto the counter. Now pick up one of the quarters and place it into your mouth; now begin to slowly suck out the lemon juice.

I then ask the audience what they feel and inevitably they remark that their mouths have begun to water—yours might have as well from merely reading the paragraph. Think about this for a moment: The mere thought of sucking on a lemon can cause your mouth to salivate. A thought purposely brought into your mind can cause a definitive physiological response in your body; in other words, you can, in effect, control the way you feel simply by the thoughts that you bring into your head. This has incredible implications when it comes to sports performance. What you should begin to do is harness this mind/body connection to better your times and have a better time during your triathlons as well as your training sessions.

Once again, self-talk is a complex subject that we will condense down for your use as a 12-Week Triathlete. Some of the uses for self-talk include:

1. Building and developing self-efficacy
2. Skill acquisition or improvement
3. Creating and changing mood
4. Controlling effort
5. Focusing attention and concentration

These may sound complicated, but you will see that they are, in fact, quite simple. You will also most likely realize that you already engage in self-talk without having really consciously thought about it. The goal now it to harness the power of self-talk.

When creating your self-talk statements, you should make them:

1. *Short and concise.* Not paragraphs long; one word or a few sentences, maximum.
2. *Positive.* This seems obvious, but many people focus on the negative.
3. *In the present tense.* "I am" rather than "I will." For example, "I feel great" rather than "I will feel great," regardless of how you actually feel at that particular moment.

Self-talk statements that rhyme work well, and you can even use song lyrics. Here are some examples of possible self-talk statements:

1. *Building and developing self-efficacy:* Self-efficacy is defined as "beliefs in one's capabilities to organize and execute the courses of action required to produce given attainments." Belief in oneself. These statements are especially useful in the days and hours leading up to your race.
   - "I can finish the swim"
   - "I am ready"
   - "I can"
2. *Skill acquisition:* Learning and bettering a particular sport skill.
   - "Reach" (during your swim stroke)
   - "Drop the heels" (during your pedal stroke)
   - "Soft feet" (during the run)
3. *Creating and changing mood:* Bringing yourself to your personal optimal level of arousal. These statements can be the most varied as they include anything that changes your mood state. They can be extremely simple yet elicit powerful feelings.
   - "I feel great!"
   - "It's a beautiful day!" (U2 song lyrics)

4. *Controlling effort:* These statements are very important to athletes, whether we need to decrease or increase our efforts. There are times during the race when adrenaline will be high, such as the swim start, and you will want to go out faster than you should. This is a great time to use self-talk statements to control your effort and pull back.

- "Slow"
- "Glide"
- "Nice and easy"

There will also be times when you will want to increase your effort; perhaps you have set a time goal of going less than two hours for your triathlon, and as you come into sight of the finish line, the clock reads "1:59:10." You then might use the following statements:

- "Hammer"
- "Pick it up"
- "Kick it in"

5. *Focusing attention and concentration:* All of the previously described self-talk statements can be used to focus your attention and concentration. All self-talk statements that help you find your personal "zone" should be stored in your mind and called upon when you need them. Again, these statements can be anything, the only stipulation is that they bring about the response in your body that you are attempting to achieve.

One of the most applicable uses of self-talk for us as triathletes comes when we are not feeling so hot during a race. The great thing about self-talk is that you can combine the concepts to achieve several things at once. For instance, let's say you have a bad side cramp during the beginning of your run leg. You may use a self-talk statement that focuses on a skill improvement, such as "Relax the shoulders." This one statement will, in effect, serve two distinct purposes.

First, you will be improving your running economy and therefore your overall performance by improving a component of your running style. Second, by doing this, you will shift your focus away from the pain, thereby eliminating the negative feeling from your consciousness.

If it seems like I spent a great deal of time on the mental side of your triathlon training, you are right, as I believe these simple concepts are so crucial to your race performance and enjoyment. The thoughts you bring into your head can truly change the way your body feels. No matter how bad I feel during a race, I tell myself I feel great, and my body responds in kind. Come up with a handful of self-talk statements to use before and during your race and practice controlling your thoughts. Do so, and I guarantee that you will go faster and have a much better time while racing as well.

★ **SMILE**

Try smiling during your race—the mere act of doing so also elicits a positive change in your body. I realized early on that it is profoundly difficult to hold a big smile on your face while thinking negative thoughts. And, yes, you can work at high intensities and perform at high levels while smiling—just watch Natascha Badmann, multiple Hawaii Ironman winner, race if you question this point. The smile will also bring about positive changes in you physiologically, which will translate into a better race performance. The worse I feel during a race, the bigger my smile.

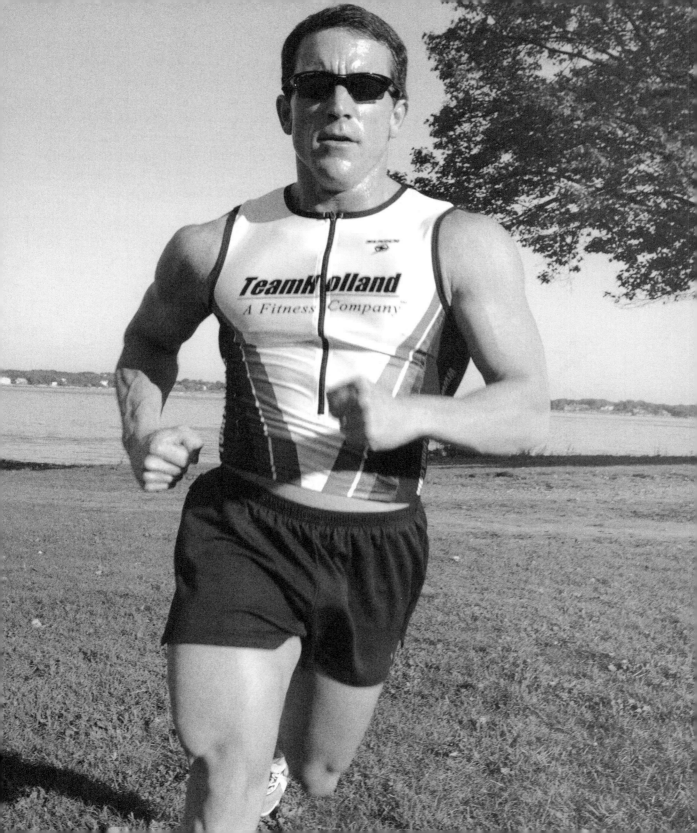

CHAPTER 11
Nutrition and Hydration

As I write this, I am a member of PowerBar's TeamElite, an age-grouper incentive-based sponsorship program. While I do receive PowerBar products for free, I absolutely believe in their value to my racing and recovery. You should experiment and determine what products work best for you.

The longer the distance of your triathlon, the more crucial to your performance as well as to your enjoyment of the event your nutrition becomes. Anyone who has ever truly "bonked" during a race can tell you that it is not a pleasant experience.

I must begin by stating that, in my experience, nutrition as it applies to sports performance in general and triathlon in particular is extremely individualized. Just like your aero position on the bike or your particular running style, what one athlete eats before and during a race might not necessarily work for you at all. One person may have a banana and toast several hours before a race, another person may eat oatmeal and an energy bar, while another may not be able to tolerate anything the morning of her event. This seems to apply to nutrition as well as hydration. I have met some who simply cannot stand the consistency of energy gels during a race—the mere thought of attempting to swallow one makes them choke. Likewise, certain brands of sports drinks do not seem to sit well for some, even certain flavors may cause stomach upset. Just like your bike fit or your running gait, there are indeed certain basic rules that apply, but in the end it comes down to your personal experimentation during training and racing. It is a never-ending process, the tweaking of all of these elements, and your nutrition is no different. In this chapter I will outline the basics of sports nutrition, but the onus is on you to take this information and find your personal prerace and race-day menu. In this chapter, I will discuss the possible options you have available to fuel yourself during your triathlons, the "whats" and "whys" of your nutrition. In the chapter on racing, I will go into greater detail on the "hows"; that is, specific strategies for nutrition and hydration.

As I write this, the low-carbohydrate diet is all the rage. Without debating the pros and cons of the resurgence of this fad diet, I can tell you unequivocally that, for us triathletes, carbs are our best friend.

Carbohydrates provide us with our main source of energy as endurance athletes. At mild intensity of exercise, fat and carbohydrate utilization is almost equal with protein, providing only a tiny percentage of energy. As intensity increases, however, carbohydrates become our primary energy source, and their depletion is what will eventually lead to our slowing down and eventually bonking. Carbohydrate is stored in our muscles and liver as glycogen, roughly 2,000 calories worth. We also have a small amount, around 80 calories, circulating in our blood in the form of glucose.

Fat is stored in our bodies in the form of triglycerides. A person with a body weight of 143 pounds and 12 percent body fat has roughly 2,000 calories stored in his liver and muscles and approximately 70,000 calories stored in his adipose tissue.

With all this potential energy in the form of fat, why do we bonk? Can't we just dip into these fat reserves? Well, the simple answer is no, our body simply cannot break down and utilize fat as readily and as effectively as it can carbohydrate. This is why it is so crucial that we have sufficient carbohydrate stores prior to our triathlons and take in additional carbohydrate during our longer-distance races.

My father began running marathons in the 1970s and completed well over a dozen without ever taking in any nutrition during these races. It just wasn't done; semisolid energy gels like PowerGels had not yet been invented when he first started running, and their incredible value to performance had not been realized and documented. It took a considerable amount of prodding, but eventually I convinced him to try several during one of his long training runs—he was amazed at the noticeable difference it made in how he felt at the later stages of these runs. He has since been converted and is running strong into his sixties with the aid of his additional carbohydrate fuel.

Again, our bodies can store roughly 2,000 calories worth of carbohydrates. The caloric expenditure obviously varies on a variety of factors, but it is believed that many who bonk at around mile 20 of a marathon do so because they have expended in the neighborhood of 600 calories per hour, and are thus almost out of energy after having exercised for three to four hours continuously. This is why it is crucial to supplement your energy stores during a marathon, and any race lasting approximately two or more hours, for that matter.

There are numerous ways to take in calories during your race: liquid, semisolid, and solid forms. Once again, a great deal of how you decide to take in your nutrition comes down to your personal experimentation. Research has shown, however, and many coaches believe, that you should try to take in the majority of your calories in semisolid and liquid form. Some say up to 80 percent of your race-day nutrition should be taken in this form. Unlike solids, semisolids and liquids are converted into usable energy more quickly and will therefore provide more effective fueling for your working muscles.

How many calories should I take in during my triathlon?

This number varies due to a variety of factors, but generally it is believed that you should try to take in 250 to 500 calories per hour during your race. Some people are on the low end of this range whereas others need more calories and perform better at the higher end. Your race distance, body size, climate, and intensity are just a few factors that may dictate your hourly caloric needs. Experiment, experiment, experiment, and find what works best for you.

One formula to determine daily caloric needs (to maintain body weight) is 30 calories per kilogram body weight.

So, 150 lb person/2.2 = 68 kilograms × 30 = 2040 calories.

Add in several hundred more calories if you are active. The more active you are, the more calories you will need to add in. Some top endurance athletes take in over 5,000 calories per day while in heavy training.

Each individual will need to experiment to determine both their caloric needs and ability to tolerate these calories while biking and running.

HYDRATION

Let's keep it simple; you need to take in fluids during your triathlon. Once again, the longer the distance, the more crucial this simple fact becomes. I would argue that, in any long-distance triathlon, a significant number of participants are suffering from some level of dehydration. It is difficult to take in as much fluid as we need; we need to follow a set schedule, drinking frequently, often drinking when we are not thirsty. Remember, once you are thirsty, it is often too late, you are already dehydrated. Your performance will suffer and you will not feel your best for the remainder of the race. Hydration is a subtle yet crucial aspect of your race strategy.

During the bike leg of Ironman Germany, I followed one particular biker (three bike lengths back, obeying the drafting rules!) for more than an hour. During this time, I watched as the two bike bottles mounted behind him stayed completely full—he never once reached back and drank from them. As I eventually pulled up to pass him, I told him that I had noticed that he was not taking in any fluids. He thanked me profusely, grabbed a bottle, and began gulping down the contents. We often get caught up in the race and "forget" to drink; you must get in the habit during your training to effectively implement your hydration schedule on race day.

Water

There is some argument as to when you should drink water and when you should drink a carbohydrate/electrolyte drink such as Gatorade during exercise. Many say that, in exercise lasting less than one hour, water is all you really need. If you are going to compete in sprint-distance triathlons and finish in just over an hour, then you may find that water is indeed all you require. My theory is this, however; we essentially need three things during our triathlons as far as nutrition and hydration: energy (carbohydrate), fluids, and electrolytes. These are three things that we either use or lose during the race. If we can get all three of these in one beverage, doesn't it make sense to do so? I believe it does. I personally drink Gatorade during all workouts, even one-hour bike rides and one-hour runs. First, I believe that these elements not found in plain water, especially the electrolyte sodium, help my training performance and recovery; second, I drink it to get my body accustomed to exactly what I plan on doing come race day.

ELECTROLYTES

The textbook definition is "a dissolved substance that can conduct electrical current." Sodium, potassium, magnesium, and chloride are all electrolytes; these enable nerve impulses to control muscle activity and also are

SALTY SWEATERS

When you finish a run in hot temperatures, (a) is there a white residue on your clothing, or (b) does your sweat taste salty as it runs into your mouth? If so, you are what is referred to as a "salty sweater" and may be losing significant sodium through your sweat. You need to be more conscious of and experiment with your sodium intake before, during, and after races and workouts.

responsible for maintaining the body's water balance, two really important things to us as triathletes. We lose electrolytes in our sweat, and significant losses can severely impair performance. One of the potential causes of muscle cramps is sodium depletion. There is still debate as to which electrolytes are most important to us as athletes, which ones potentially need to be replaced during exercise. Many now contend that sodium plays the most crucial role and therefore may need to be added to one's diet prerace and taken in during longer races as well. Let's be honest; most Americans take in significant amounts of sodium in their daily diets, especially those who consume a great deal of processed foods. If you are one of these people, you may not need to take in additional sodium prior to your race. If you do not have a diet that contains a great deal of sodium, however, you may need to preload as well as consume electrolyte drinks or take salt tablets during your long-distance triathlon.

Check with your doctor before adding sodium to your diet.

LIQUID NUTRITION
Gatorade
One of the easiest and most effective ways to get in your nutrition and hydration is through an electrolyte/carbohydrate beverage such as Gatorade. Gatorade not only supplies you with much-needed carbohydrate for energy, but it also provides you with your fluids as well as electrolytes (see discussion on electrolytes above). Gatorade and Gatorade-like drinks are usually provided at the aid stations during most races.

Twenty ounces of lemon-lime flavored, the amount that would fill one regular-sized bike bottle, contains 125 calories and ingredients including:
Sodium: 330 mg
Potassium: 90 mg
Carbohydrate: 35 g
Protein: 0 g

So, for shorter-distance triathlons, if you are racing for just over an hour, say, you can get all or the majority of your fluids and calories in through a drink like Gatorade. One full bike bottle of a Gatorade-type beverage will give you about 125 calories of fuel.

PowerBar's Beverage System
PowerBar has developed a new "Beverage System," including their own version of Gatorade, PowerBar Endurance sport drink, along with a PowerBar Performance Recovery drink for after exercise. They developed this system

with Chris Carmichael, Lance Armstrong's coach. In the Performance Recovery drink they include a small amount of protein.

Twenty ounces of PowerBar Endurance sport drink, for use during exercise, contains the following:

Calories: 175
Sodium: 400 mg
Potassium: 25 mg
Carbohydrate: 42.5 g
Protein: 0 g
Magnesium: 4%
Chloride: 2 %

Twenty ounces of PowerBar Recovery, for postexercise, contains the following:

Calories: 225
Sodium: 625 mg
Potassium: 25 mg
Carbohydrate: 50 g
Protein: 7.5 g
Magnesium: 4%
Chloride: 6%

Ensure

As you get into the Half-Ironman and Ironman-distance races, you may find you need more

⭐ **HYPONATREMIA**

A condition that arises during endurance events that can potentially be fatal, hyponatremia is due to abnormally low sodium levels in the body. It is often caused by a variety of factors, but the main culprit is drinking excessive amounts of water prior to, and during an endurance event. Taking in too much plain water flushes the sodium from your body, lowering it to potentially dangerous levels in the presence of other conditions. It occurs more often in women, in those who consume large quantities of water prerace, in those who take NSAIDs (nonsteroidal anti-inflammatory drugs), in those who continue to drink large amounts of water during the race without replacing electrolytes, and in those who remain out on the course for long periods of time. While still relatively uncommon in races, it is something to consider when racing longer-distance triathlons, especially the Ironman. Several studies have focused on the number of athletes suffering from this condition at the end of the Hawaii Ironman, and more recently, twelve runners were treated for hyponatremia at the 2004 Boston Marathon. Even though the chances of experiencing hyponatremia may be low, it is a concern of many race directors today, and you should be aware of the conditions that may cause it. The best way to avoid hyponatremia during long events is to be sure to consume an electrolyte beverage such as Gatorade during your race. These beverages will provide you with the fluid as well as the electrolytes your body needs to function optimally, especially in hot conditions.

calories than Gatorade can provide or that you can tolerate from Gatorade alone. I use, and recommend that my clients try, a high-calorie liquid supplement such as Ensure. Ensure is extremely calorie dense, especially Ensure Plus.

One 8-ounce bottle of vanilla flavored Ensure Plus contains the following ingredients:

Calories: 360
Sodium: 240 mg
Potassium: 440 mg
Carbohydrate: 50 g
Fat: 11 g
Protein: 13 g

For my Ironman races, I personally carry one 20-ounce bike bottle filled with Ensure Plus. This is my major source of calories. It translates into roughly 875 calories, 125 grams of carbohydrate, and a good amount of sodium.

SEMISOLID NUTRITION

Many people now refer to semisolid nutrition by the brand name of one specific product, Gu. Pronounced like goo, it is a gel-like substance that tastes like it sounds and has a similar consistency

as well. There are, in fact, many different brands and flavors of gels on the market today, including PowerBar's PowerGels, which I use and recommend because they provide much needed and easily digestible fuel in the form of carbohydrate. Gels primarily come in single-serving packets, little foil squares that hold this gooey mixture, which you tear open during a race. It is suggested that you take the gel with water. You now can carry the gel in special flasks that attach to your bike, or in bottles that you wear during the run on a special belt made for this very purpose.

PowerBar's PowerGels

One packet of Tangerine-flavor PowerGel contains ingredients including:

Calories: 110
Sodium: 45 mg
Potassium: 45 mg
Chloride: 90 mg
Carbohydrate: 26 g

SOLID NUTRITION

When we think of solid nutrition during a race, we generally are referring to energy bars, but it is by no means limited to bars alone. Fruit, candy, pretzels; the sky's the limit as to what some people eat during their triathlons. The key is to find energy that fuels you and that you can "stomach" during a race. I know of some athletes who have a peanut butter and jelly sandwich in their Bento Box that they eat during their Ironman races. Others stock their "special needs" bags (more on these in the chapter on racing) with a small convenience store of food items. When we think of solid nutrition, however, most likely it will be a type of energy bar that you carry with you on the bike. Remember that you generally want to try to take in the majority of your calories in liquid or semisolid form; some athletes find, however, that they need a little solid food to achieve a comfortable feeling in their stomach while racing. During the bike leg some keep an energy bar in their bike jersey, in a fanny pack, in a Bento Box, or even cut into pieces and "molded" onto their top tube, to be pulled off as they bike.

Once again, during the longer-distance triathlons, energy bars and solid foods are often provided. Research what brands and flavors will be on the course and practice using them during your training if you plan on taking them in on race day.

Energy Bars

Here is the breakdown of two popular energy bars that you may work into your overall nutritional strategy:

PowerBar Performance: Peanut Butter Flavor
Calories: 240
Sodium: 120 mg
Potassium: 130 mg
Carbohydrate: 45 g
Protein: 10 g

Clif Bar: Chocolate Chip Peanut Crunch
Calories: 250
Sodium: 210 mg
Potassium: 220 mg
Carbohydrate: 43 g
Protein: 11 g

★ CARBOHYDRATE AND PROTEIN

Recent research is indicating that it is advantageous to take carbohydrate and protein together to optimally replenish glycogen stores and make energy more readily available for our use—the protein may play an important role in how our bodies "uptake" the carbohydrate. More and more products are coming onto the market now that are incorporating this science and that have this mix of carbs and protein, for use both during the race and for recovery postrace and postworkout. Many also now believe that you may want this small amount of protein during exercise as well. A ratio of 4:1 carbs to protein is often cited in the research; PowerBar's Recovery drink contains roughly a 7:1 ratio, and Ensure has about a 5:1 ratio.

FUEL ON THE GO

It is advisable to try to get the majority of your calories in during the bike leg rather than during the run. Most people will find they can tolerate taking in more calories when they are supported on a bike rather than while they are running.

B.Y.O.N.—BRING YOUR OWN NUTRITION

Don't ever rely on getting food on the course; always have a backup plan, and whenever possible, try to carry your most important items with you. For example, even though the race information states that chocolate Ironman bars will be given out at all aid stations, they can and often do run out of these items as the race progresses. If you were depending on that 250 calories and have nothing with you, your performance will suffer. Bring as much with you as you can.

FUELING DURING THE RUN

Depending on the distance of your triathlon and the food on the course, you may have to carry additional calories with you during the run. Yet again, you should have practiced this during your training, and you should simply have to follow the same strategy you utilized during your longer run workouts. Semisolids such as PowerGels are great for Half-Ironman and Ironman-distance races. I recommend clients premix the PowerGels with water and carry them in their Fuel Belts. You are supposed to take these gels with liquid—by using this strategy, you can take the gel exactly when you need to instead of waiting for an aid station.

My current strategy is that I premix two PowerGels in each Fuel Belt bottle and drink half the bottle (one PowerGel) every half hour during the Ironman run.

Okay, I understand my nutritional options for my race, but how should I eat during my training?

This is one of the most frequently asked questions—what type of day-to-day diet should be followed during your triathlon training. I believe that a healthy daily diet for a normal person is not markedly different from the one you should follow as a triathlete, the only difference being that you need to eat more to compensate for all the calories you are burning. It's a great thing, being a triathlete! People always are astonished at how much I eat, but I have to fuel my workouts as well as recover from them. Good eating is not as much about deprivation as it is about healthy choices, in my experience. I believe that the following basic guidelines comprise the outline of a great healthy diet plan:

1. Eat approximately every three hours; five to six medium-sized meals a day.
2. Eat whole foods: fruits, vegetables, complex carbohydrates, and good lean sources of protein.
3. Drink lots of water.
4. Eat or drink a recovery meal as close to workouts as possible.

Simple, yet the successful formulas usually are! Like your triathlon training itself, it's the consistent application of the principles that is difficult and the key to success, not the complexity of the program itself.

Obviously, you may have to take in a recovery meal earlier than your scheduled meal that falls every three hours. This is okay, and it is more important that you take that food in as

★ THE RECOVERY MEAL

What is the benefit to eating or drinking a recovery meal immediately following a workout? Recent research indicates that there is a "metabolic window," a period of approximately forty-five minutes immediately after a workout, when your body can optimally replenish and rebuild itself. Again, it seems as if a carbohydrate and protein mix works best, in a ratio of about 4:1 carbohydrate to protein. The body is best able to "restock" your glycogen (carb) stores and begin to rebuild the muscle broken down during exercise at this time. The more frequently and the more intensely you work out, the more crucial it is that you replace your energy stores in preparation for your next session. There are numerous products on the market for just this purpose, recovery, including the PowerBar drink by that name as well as Endurox, another popular brand used by triathletes.

OTHER POSSIBLE RECOVERY MEALS:
1. Pasta and tuna
2. Wheat bread with peanut butter
3. Pasta with chicken
4. Brown rice and beans
5. A power shake: frozen fruit with protein powder

close to completing your workout as possible rather than waiting several hours for your next meal. Try to time your workouts and eating plan as best as you can, but life often gets in the way and steers us off schedule. I try to take in a recovery drink rather than a meal if I complete a workout before my next scheduled meal. I do not count this recovery drink as one of my six meals of the day. I try to eat carbohydrate and protein together at all meals.

SAMPLE DAILY EATING PLAN

7 AM: Oatmeal and power shake

10 AM: Egg-white omelette with vegetables and whole wheat toast

1 PM: Tuna on a garden salad

3 PM: Fruit salad and peanut butter on whole wheat bread

6 PM: Chicken with brown rice and vegetables

9 PM: Energy bar

★ **MY MORNING POWER SHAKE**

I mix the following ingredients in a blender for a healthy and great-tasting carbohydrate-and-protein breakfast drink.

1. Protein powder
2. Water
3. Splash of orange juice
4. Flaxseed oil
5. Banana
6. Frozen fruit (strawberries, blueberries, mixed berries, etc.)

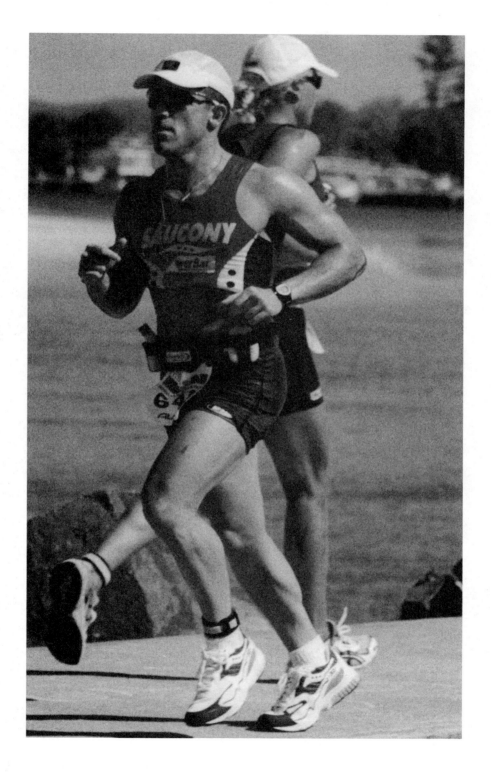

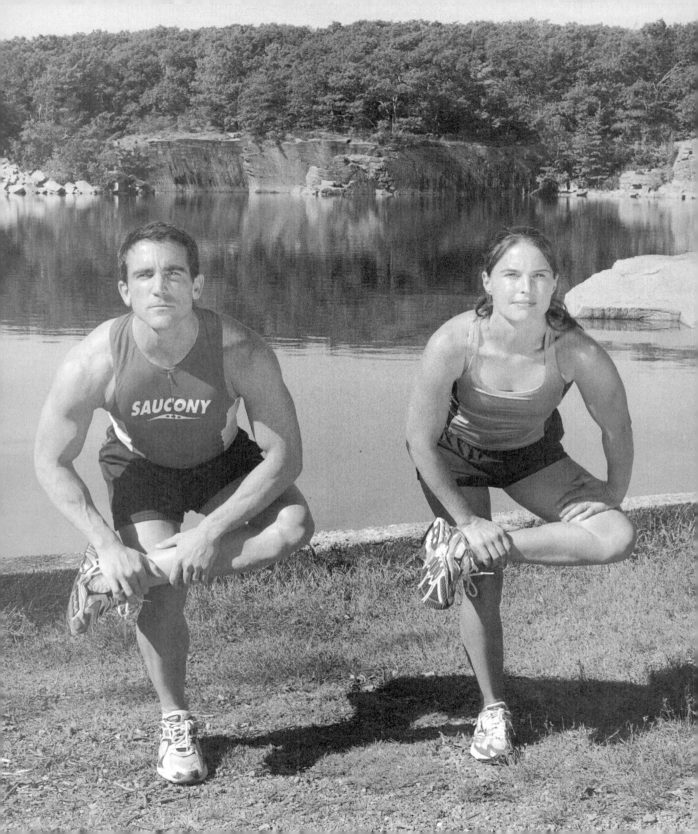

CHAPTER 12

Prerace Considerations

During the two weeks prior to your triathlon, in your Taper Phase, there are certain things that you should do to prepare for your race. As some of you will be competing in triathlons at home whereas others will travel to their races and arrive a week or more in advance, what these preparations are and exactly when you do them will change somewhat as a result. What I will outline, therefore, are the basics that you should follow as they apply to your particular race situation.

WEEK 10: THE TAPER BEGINS

Two weeks until race day; your Taper begins. You may look at the schedule and think that it does not look like enough training given what you have been doing for the past two and a half months. Or perhaps you breathe a sign of relief while looking forward to the added rest and more free time on the weekends. Realize this and take it to heart: I believe that a large percentage of athletes sabotage their training in the Taper Phase. They simply cannot or will not pull back their training. They either continue to train at equal volume or even try to "cram" training in, adding in additional workouts and increasing the length of workouts as well. This is not like studying for a test at the last minute—training hard during your taper will only serve to hurt your performance come race day. It is during the Taper Phase that your body is allowed

to truly "take in" all of the training that you have been engaging in, recovering and rebuilding so that you can fire off of that start line on race morning. You will be engaging in shorter workouts, which by no means will be diminishing your race day performance; in fact, this is essential in bringing it about. If you have truly trained consistently up to this point, I would argue that you could almost take these two weeks off completely and you would still have a great race. Less is more now. Quality over quantity. Go too hard during your Taper Phase and you will toe that start line fatigued, possibly injured, with less-than-optimal energy stores and dead legs.

TEST-RUN TRIATHLON

Although this will not be specifically included in the 12-Week Triathlete training schedules, two weeks out from your race is a great time to stage a short "mock triathlon." Basically, you will practice your transitions to work out any kinks and see what works and what doesn't. As always, the closer you can duplicate your race-day conditions, the better. So, you would go to the beach or the pool to begin, bringing all of your race clothing and gear with you. You needn't swim more than a few minutes in your race clothing, then exit the water and change into your biking gear. Not to beat a dead horse, but once again you need to do this exactly the

"STOP, DROP, AND PULL"

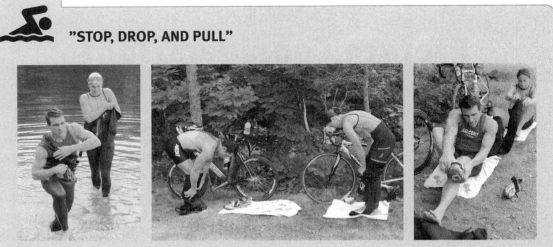

"Stop…"   "drop…"   "…and pull!"

There is a certain technique to removing your wetsuit. When you have finished swimming and are walking out of the water, you can unzip your wetsuit, take out your arms and pull it down around your waist. Leave it there as you jog to your transition area.

Once you arrive at your transition area, immediately drop to your butt on the ground, then pull your wetsuit down your legs with both hands. It's almost impossible to remove your wetsuit while standing; you end up bouncing around, trying to balance on one leg, then come crashing down when you inevitably lose your balance. The technique is kind of a modification of what you are supposed to do if you're on fire, except instead of "Stop, drop, and roll," it's "Stop, drop, and pull."

Don't make the same mistake I did during my first Half-Ironman in Florida. The swim was in the Gulf and I had been taught the above-mentioned technique several weeks earlier by a top triathlon coach. Eager to try it out and shave a few seconds from my transition time, as soon as I got close enough to shore to stand, I did so and quickly pulled my wetsuit down to my waist. Turns out I did this a little too early—as I jogged through the water and was a few dozen yards from shore, the ocean floor dropped out and I was forced to swim once again. The wetsuit now acted like an anchor as I flopped around like a wounded seal for the last few yards to shore. This small mistake ended up costing me additional time, energy, and frustration. Make sure you are truly in walking distance to shore before trying this wetsuit removal strategy!

way you plan to race. In other words, if you want to wear a certain necklace or bandanna during your triathlon, you need to try it out during the test run, because you may discover that this important necklace causes you incredible grief during your swim or that wearing a bandanna under your bike helmet makes it too tight and gives you a headache.

This "dry run" should also be considered a "wet run," because simple transition elements can change due to something like your being wet from the swim.

A client of mine who was participating in her first triathlon had done all of her pre-race preparations except for staging a little mock triathlon to practice her transitions. Well, she started her race with a great swim, then emerged from the water and sprinted to her transition area. As she attempted to pull her bike top on, she discovered that this simple task was now exponentially more difficult due to her wet skin. The shirt was stuck like glue on her shoulders, and she fought with it for a good couple of minutes before she was finally able to pull it down. Had she tried this in practice, she would have uncovered this "sticking point" and devised a new technique for pulling that bike jersey on.

This point is especially true when it comes to wetsuit removal. At the bigger triathlons, they actually often have volunteer "strippers," people whose sole job it is to pull your wetsuit off of you as you emerge from the water. This volunteer job exists because it can be extremely difficult to take a wetsuit off in normal circumstances, not to mention during race conditions, when you will be somewhat disoriented from the swim and full of adrenaline. So, if you will be using a wetsuit during

your triathlon and will be taking it off yourself, be sure to practice doing so at this time.

DESTINATION TRIATHLONS

For those of you who will be flying to your triathlons, you will obviously have to transport your bike, and this is a science in and of itself. What you need to think about:

1. *A bike box:* You need to carry your bike in something. There are plain old cardboard boxes used to ship new bikes to the bike store. This is the cheapest option and the chances of your bike arriving intact to your destination are not very good. Then there are hard cases made specifically for protecting bikes being shipped by air. These are not cheap; they cost around $250 to $500 for a good one. If you plan to travel with your bike often, then this might be a good investment. Many bike stores also rent these cases, and you can always see if a friend of yours will lend you one. I often lend mine to my friend Nick, who is an incredible cyclist but also incredibly cheap. You will put your wheels in the box and whatever else you can fit in, such as bike shoes, pump, wetsuit, et cetera.

2. *Shipping your bike:* Consider shipping your bike by a service such as FedEx or UPS. Shipping your bike ahead of time can save a lot of headaches: It can actually be cheaper, you won't have to drag your bike through airports and pay for oversize rental cars, and your bike won't get lost as many bikes do when they fly with their owners. You do not want to arrive in St. Croix and discover that your

bike is now in Paris! At every triathlon I have traveled to, I have watched numerous athletes stand in silent horror at the baggage claim waiting in vain for their bikes to appear. Check out the costs and time frame associated with shipping your bike directly to your hotel or wherever you are staying.

3. *Airline costs:* Most airlines will charge you to take a bike with you on board. The cost of taking your bike with you on the plane can range from nothing to $100, and I have yet to pay the same price twice for this service. Don't be surprised at the ticket counter with this unforeseen cost; check your airline's policy on bikes as baggage ahead of time. This alone may convince you to ship it in advance.

4. *Disassembly/assembly:* When shipping your bike, you will most likely have to take it apart to fit it into your bike case. The handlebars will need to come off, both of the pedals, and the seat. If you do not know how to do this or do not feel comfortable doing this, then bring it in to your local bike shop and have them pack it up for you.

   If you are willing to spend a little extra, many bike shops will pack and ship the bike for you for a fee, and you can do this both going to your triathlon and coming back home. So, you bring your bike and your bike case to your local bike shop. They pack it and ship it to the bike shop at your race destination (most big races have bike shops that serve as the "official bike shop" of the triathlon). This bike shop will then receive your bike, set

it up, and tune it so it is ready to go when you arrive. When you leave, you simply reverse the process. It may cost a few extra dollars to send it by this method, but if it is available to you, I believe this is by far the best way to go.

5. *Carry important gear on the plane:* Bikes get lost and luggage gets lots as well. Don't make the mistake of having a bag lost that contains items or gear that you cannot race without and may not be able to replace at the race site.

6. *CO2 cartridges:* If you use CO2 cartridges, remember that airlines will not allow these to be carried in your baggage, not even your checked luggage. At some of the smaller airports associated with bigger triathlons, they even check your luggage specifically for these if you tell them you are a triathlete. As I was leaving St. Croix after competing in the triathlon, the baggage checker had a box full of confiscated CO2 cartridges. Now, I know many people send them anyway, and I am a firm believer in bringing everything you need with you, but you can purchase these at the race expo or from the local bike shop. Don't waste your money buying CO2s that will only be taken from you and could potentially be hazardous on the flight.

Do not ever bring your bike tools in your carry-on luggage. The airlines now confiscate all "tools" seemingly regardless of their ability to be used as a potential weapon. I recently made this mistake and had all of my bike tools taken from me during my trip to Ironman South Korea.

SWIM

Your swim sessions should now be done in exactly what you will be wearing on race day. Let me reiterate that: exactly.

If you will be wearing a wetsuit, you should get accustomed to it for at least several swims, especially if you have never used one before, wearing underneath it what you will wear race morning. If you plan on wearing anything like a heart rate monitor, wear it during these swims as well. You will be shocked at how some things fit or feel, rub or chafe, that you did not expect—you do not want to find this out during your race. If you plan on buying new goggles, do so now, and make sure they fit and work for you. I recommend purchasing two pairs if possible, in case something happens to one.

Wetsuit and the Pool

Perhaps your triathlon will be in the open water and you will be wearing a wetsuit, but you do not have the opportunity to train in the open water. I still recommend that you swim at least several times in the wetsuit, even in the pool. You need to become accustomed to the feel of swimming in a wetsuit before your race, making sure it fits properly as well and has no major defects. Some people may feel self-conscious about putting on a wetsuit and swimming in a public pool—I say, who cares what the other swimmers think? You are the one who will be swimming in the wetsuit during your triathlon, and you will gain added peace of mind as well as performance benefits from having trained in it.

BIKE TUNE-UP

It's a good idea to have your bike tuned up roughly two weeks before your race. This gives you enough time to deal with any major issues that may be found during the tune-up, in case any new parts need to be ordered or replaced. If you are knowledgeable in bike maintenance, then this would be a good time to perform the tune-up yourself as well. I leave the tune-ups to the professionals at my local bike shop, getting a complete overhaul done. It can be expensive, but the bike is the one thing during your triathlon that can break down and prevent you from finishing your race. The money spent is well worth it, in my opinion, especially given all the time and money you have already invested. I have seen triathletes' races come to an end because of a fifty-cent part that was worn down and then broke during the bike leg. Having a qualified bike mechanic check over your bike gives you one less thing to worry about as your race approaches.

Now is also a good time to make sure that you have all of your gear and that it is all in proper working order. There is nothing worse than waking up race morning and realizing that you forgot to replace your broken goggles, buy spare tubes, buy your nutrition, et cetera. If a store is out of your particular brand or flavor of something, you still have adequate time to find it. I would have everything assembled two weeks prior to your triathlon so that your equipment is one less thing that you have to worry about.

If you do plan on buying anything like a new helmet, new bike shoes, or a new race outfit, do it now so that you can try everything out in training first. This goes for everything; new running shoes, tri shorts, bike jerseys, hats, sunglasses, everything. Buy it now and test it all out in at least one workout, preferably two or more.

★ TRIATHLON CHECKLIST

I am including everything in the following checklist; you will not necessarily need or use all of the items for your particular race. You may also have a few additional items that you will be using—make sure those are ready to go as well. Remember that it is better to bring too much and not use a few items than to kick yourself for not bringing something on race morning.

SWIM
- ☐ Swimsuit
- ☐ 2 sets of goggles (one just in case)
- ☐ Towels
- ☐ Wetsuit

BIKE
- ☐ Bike (tuned up)
- ☐ Helmet
- ☐ Sunglasses
- ☐ Bike jersey
- ☐ Bike shorts
- ☐ Socks
- ☐ Gloves
- ☐ Water bottles
- ☐ Bike nutrition: liquid/gel/solid
- ☐ 2 spare tubes or tubulars
- ☐ Bike shoes
- ☐ Bike tool
- ☐ 2 tire levers
- ☐ Bike-mounted bike pump
  or CO2 cartridges and valve
- ☐ Floor pump

RUN
- ☐ Running shoes
- ☐ Socks
- ☐ Run shorts
- ☐ Run shirt
- ☐ Run nutrition: liquid/gel/solid
- ☐ Hat

OTHER
- ☐ Watch
- ☐ Race belt
- ☐ Fuel Belt
- ☐ Sunscreen
- ☐ Body Glide
- ☐ Band-Aids/Liquid Bandage/Vaseline
- ☐ Assorted types of tape (you never know)
- ☐ Water
- ☐ Snacks

Do not wait until the last minute to buy any of these products. Purchase and assemble together everything you need; the last thing you want is to be scrambling all over town trying to find something at the last minute. This situation does not help in getting you to your optimal state of arousal.

WEEK 11: SECOND WEEK OF THE TAPER

Most likely you are ready to pull your hair out now. You are tired and cranky. You can't believe it, but you actually miss some of those workouts you dreaded just several weeks ago. Your legs feel heavy during your bikes and runs, and you feel as if you are swimming through molasses in the pool.

This is normal.

This is the time to turn to your journal and start reading it. Begin with week one and work your way slowly through each consecutive week, noting all of the hours and miles you have logged in your training. See the improvements that you have inevitably made and probably forgot about. Remember all those really tough workouts that you did not want to do but you suffered through anyway. If you have been relatively consistent with your training, then reading your journal should really add to your confidence level. Many people are in the best shape of their lives as they approach the race day of their first triathlon—chances are you are now in really great shape as well. Take pride in all of the sacrifices you have made, how disciplined you have been, and what great things you have done for your health.

The "Triathlon Stress Dreams"

If they didn't start several weeks ago, they most likely will begin to haunt you now. In them, you are at your triathlon when something inevitably goes wrong. They can range from typical to the surreal to the bizarre: You are traveling by plane and your bike gets lost, you forget to put your helmet in your transition area, you oversleep, you take a wrong turn on the bike course, and so on. I have had my share of TSDs, my favorite being the one where I exit the swim and run to the transition area. Everything else is normal except that, instead of bikes, the transition area is full of horses, and I can't find mine. Everyone else is galloping out of T1 as I run in circles trying to locate my horse.... It seems that no one is immune from these nighttime experiences—I would bet good money that the top professional triathletes have them as well.

Concentrate on your visualization and your relaxation exercises now to help alleviate anxiety. Picture yourself having a great race, enjoying every moment, feeling strong from beginning to end. Add in additional relaxation exercise sessions.

Your body is adjusting to the reduced volume of training and these are the common symptoms. Do not give in to the temptation to deviate from the program and add in additional workouts. You cannot improve your cardiovascular system with your workouts in these final days; your workouts are maintenance and serve to keep you fresh for race day. You will not get faster, stronger, or improve your endurance in these last few days. Your most important workouts now? Rest.

As this final week progresses, you will become more and more nervous. You will feel even more tired. Cranky? Absolutely. Your whole body hurts, and the tiniest bit of soreness or tightness now will be magnified 100 times. You will feel fat. You will question your training: Did I swim enough? Did I bike enough?

Once again, welcome to the Taper.

You may really start to feel stressed now as well. Stress is obviously not a good thing, and it's something we should try to avoid. The good news is that stress is controllable; it is a choice. There is a great quote that I keep on the wall of my office that reads:

Emotion is a direct manifestation of a person's appraisal of any given situation. —Richard Lazarus

What does this mean? Translated for our purposes, it means that it is not the situation itself that is stressful; it is our perception of the situation. The triathlon is not stressful in and of itself; it is if we let it be so. Relax, the hard work is over. "Game day," the fun part, is not too far away!

CARBOHYDRATE LOADING

There is still some debate as to whether endurance athletes need to take in additional carbohydrates or "carbo load" before an event. Some coaches and exercise physiologists contend that you need not change your diet prerace. They believe that, if you taper down correctly, you will be exercising less, thus burning fewer daily calories, so you will be, in effect, carbo loading by simply eating the same diet you have been eating all along. I agree with this logic but still believe that additional carbohydrates should be taken in prior to your longer-distance triathlons.

For those of you who will be finishing your triathlons in two hours or less, this should not be an issue given a healthy diet and good recovery nutrition practices during training.

For those of you planning on racing for more than two hours, I believe you should take in additional carbohydrates. I think three days prior to your race is a good time to begin. So, if you are racing on Saturday, I would begin to increase you daily carbohydrate intake on Wednesday. Now, this is not a good time to begin experimenting with foods that you are not used to eating, so stick with healthy, carbohydrate-rich foods that you are accustomed to eating. Pastas, breads, and oatmeal are some possibilities. The goal of all this is to "top off" your energy stores, loading your muscles and liver with as much glycogen as your body can store so you have as much energy as possible available to you during your triathlon. Eating additional carbs with most meals during this period is an easy way to start preloading your body. You don't need to go overboard and gorge yourself; simply increasing the size of your meals slightly with healthy carbohydrate-rich foods should increase your glycogen reserves.

CARBOHYDRATE DRINKS

There are numerous carbohydrate drinks on the market today that you can use to take in additional quantities of carbohydrate before your triathlon. I personally use them for all my endurance events and have found them to be a simple and convenient way to carbo load before a race.

These drinks are really helpful if you will be traveling to your triathlon, especially to a foreign country where you are not sure what foods will be available to you prerace. I actually ship a case of these drinks to my destination ahead of time so that I don't have to lug them along with me when I travel.

Many of my clients have used these drinks before their races with positive results. Some choices of carbo-loading drinks include:

Ultra Fuel by TwinLab
Calories: 400
Carbohydrates: 100 g

Carbo Force by ABB
Calories: 440
Carbohydrates: 110 g

As you can see, both of these drinks are packed with calories and carbohydrates. Like anything else, you should experiment with these drinks during your training if you plan on using them before your race. If you are planning on doing a long brick workout or a long run, you can try consuming one or two of these drinks the day before and see how you feel during your long training session.

I personally drink three or four of these drinks per day for the three days prior to my long triathlons. It may seem like a lot, but it has really seemed to work for me in the energy department on race day. I have also had clients who have chosen to do the same and take in two to four of these per day for several days before their races, also with positive results.

Where did I come up with this carbo-loading strategy? A scientific journal? Am I sponsored by these companies? No—a professional triathlete at my first Ironman in New Zealand passed it along to me as it was part of his prerace preparations. His hotel room was full of these types of drinks, and he was taking them in to prepare for his race. I tried them as well, and they have worked for me ever since. Before my first ultra marathon, running 36 miles to the 10,028-foot summit of Mt. Haleakala on Maui, I employed this carbo-loading strategy yet again, with incredible results. It was the altitude that inevitably slowed me down; my energy levels stayed almost constant throughout the entire run, and I attribute a great deal of this to taking in almost a dozen of these types of drinks in the days leading up to the run. Will this strategy necessarily work for you? Maybe not. But however you achieve it, you want you body to have as much stored glycogen as possible before your long-distance triathlon.

Obviously, a great deal of how you will eat depends on the makeup of your normal daily diet. You may already eat an incredible amount of carbohydrates and thus may not need to take in as much as someone else who consumes fewer carbohydrates and total calories daily.

To summarize:
1. You will need carbohydrates as fuel for your triathlon.
2. The longer the triathlon, the more carbs you will burn and thus need.
3. Taking in more carbs than normal beginning several days prior to your race may help increase your stored levels of carbohydrate.
4. You can take in these additional carbohydrates in foods rich in complex carbohydrates and/or carbohydrate drinks.

SODIUM LOADING
Like carbohydrate loading, you may want to consider loading up on sodium (salt) during this time frame as well, especially if:
1. You sweat a great deal during exercise.
2. Your sweat often leaves a white residue on your clothing.
3. You will be participating in a long-distance triathlon.

4. Your race will be in a hot environment.
5. Your normal daily diet is low in sodium.

Remember that sodium depletion can severely impact your race performance, especially by causing painful muscle cramps. You can take in this additional salt in numerous ways, including eating foods rich in sodium, such as pretzels, consuming drinks such as V8 juice, or salting your food a little more during these few days. If you have any issues with high blood pressure, be sure to check with your doctor before increasing your sodium intake.

REGISTRATION

You need to check in for your race, and often it will be one to three days before your triathlon. Do it as soon as you can; it is yet one less thing to think about. When checking in, you will pick up your race packet, which will generally be a bag containing some or all of the following:

1. Your swim cap
2. Your race numbers, which can include:
   - Run bib number (This is pinned to the front of your shirt or worn on the front with a race belt.)
   - Bike bib number (This is pinned on the back of your shirt or worn on your back with a race belt.)
   - Number for your bike
   - Helmet number
3. Timing chip (if the race will be using this method)
4. Instructions and rules
5. Free stuff from the race sponsors
6. Transition bags (generally for Half-Ironman and Ironman races)

Read all of the instructions from start to finish. Don't skip these no matter how many triathlons you have done—each race can have its own unique rules and procedures. Read them and follow them.

When I participated in Ironman Australia, I prepared as I would for my numerous prior Ironman races. Check-in was the night before the race, where we turned in our transition bags (more on these later) and our bike. Well, at this race, they checked through all of the transition bags, not a usual occurrence at an Ironman event. They pulled out my race belt with my run number on it that I use as both my bike and run number. They asked where my bike number was, and I replied that I was just using the run number as I and so many others have done many times before. Well, it turns out that they insisted that you use both numbers as there were two different sponsors on each one and each sponsor wanted to get their money's worth with this exposure. This information had been in the race packet, which I did not read fully, and therefore I had significant stress as they put my bag aside and would not check it in without that number. I could not bring it that night, so race morning I had to scramble to find the official and give him my number, then pray that he would find my bag, put the number in, and put my bag in the appropriate place. Read everything and follow all directions.

These directions should be in your race packet, but here is a basic idea of the prerace setup of materials provided:

1. If one is provided, affix the bike number to your bike frame. It is generally placed on the top tube or seat post—this often depends on your particular bike setup.

Just make sure that it can be seen by a race official and that it does not interfere with your pedal stroke. (This is one reason you perform that last short workout with all your race gear in place—oftentimes an athlete will do something such as affix this number somewhere on the bike, only to discover during the race that it scrapes him or her somewhere and really interferes with his or her performance. This little thing can turn into a nightmare during longer races.) You will usually either affix the number with twist ties provided, or it will be a sticker that wraps around your tube. If it does require twist ties, it is a good idea to cut the excess off to avoid possible contact with your body. If it is a sticker, be sure to guesstimate where you will place it before trying to place it on as you really only have one shot to do this. Again, do not modify this number in any way, as this can often be against the rules and cause you unnecessary grief.

2. There may often be a race number sticker for your helmet. Place that in the appropriate location as specified by the directions. It is often put right on the front of your helmet.

Do these things right away and leave everything else in the bag.

THE PRERACE MEETING

Almost all races have a mandatory prerace meeting. It usually takes place the day before the event, and this is where the race rules and regulations will be discussed. Once again, do not skip this meeting, no matter how many races you have participated in. The same situation applies to the race meeting as it did to the reading of your race information packet—there are numerous topics that will be discussed at the race meeting that you need to know. Realize also that the race information packet does not always contain all the necessary race information, and many times, things are changed at the last minute—things that if you are not aware of them can really ruin your race. The race meeting is also your only real opportunity to ask questions. Yes, the meetings are often long, and yes, most of the information you will already know, but these meetings are deemed mandatory for a reason.

At my last race, almost everyone was drinking from water bottles at the prerace meeting; why, and should I be doing the same?

Yes, many triathletes show up at the prerace meeting sipping constantly from bike bottles. There are two reasons for this: One, the obvious, they are taking in additional fluids prior to the race, trying to ensure that they start their race in the morning fully hydrated. Taking in additional fluids before your race is generally a good idea, but do not overdo it—you should not take in excessive amounts of water prior to your race and potentially set yourself up for hyponatremia as a result. A few extra bike bottles full should be plenty. The second reason I believe triathletes show up with these bike bottles is anxiety—it gives them something to do. The Taper is killing them with the reduced amount of training volume, and that, coupled with the stress of the race, makes them need this "prerace pacifier." Hydrate, but do not overdo it.

THE PEACOCK PARADE

This is what I have termed the procession that occurs at triathlons the days preceding the race. At the expo, registration, prerace meeting, carbo dinner, around town, at church services—athletes will wear all of their best finisher's gear clothing from prior races, including hats, T-shirts, jackets, Speedos, you name it. They will wear the most impressive clothing from the best race they have competed in, and this often makes first-time triathletes even more nervous. Ignore it and block it out—chances are you may finish in front of many of these same people. And you'll be doing the same at your next race. Just do me a favor; if it's 90 degrees outside, please don't wear your Boston Marathon winter jacket...that's a little obvious.

TRANSITION BAGS

Transition bags are generally used in the bigger and longer triathlons, such as the Ironman-distance races. In these races you will not be setting up a transition area, you will rather be placing your gear in special bags that you will take into a changing area (often a large tent) at each transition. They include the following:

1. *Dry clothes bag:* This bag you take with you to the swim start before your race. In it you will put the clothes you wore that morning and any other items you brought with you to the race start. They will usually have a bag drop-off point somewhere close to the race start where you will put this bag after you change into your swim gear. I use this bag to carry items down with me to the race start, such as my prerace food and drinks and my filled bike bottles and Fuel Belt bottles. You will retrieve this bag at the finish line, so if you want warm clothes or other items at that point, you should also include them.

2. *Swim-to-bike bag:* This bag holds all of your biking gear: your helmet, sunglasses, gloves, jersey, shorts, shoes, socks, race number, and any other items that you may want before you begin the bike leg of your race (Vaseline, sunscreen, food items, last will and testament, etc.). As you exit the water from the swim, you will grab this bag, take it to the changing area, and dress for the bike leg, placing all of your used swim items in this bag, such as your wetsuit and goggles.

3. *Bike-to-run bag:* The same concept as the swim-to-bike bag; in here you will put all of your running gear. You will come off of the bike, get this bag, and take it into the changing area. You will remove your bike clothes (if you change for the run; many do not) and put on your run gear, placing your bike gear back in this bag. Contents of this bag may include your running shoes, run clothing, hat, sunglasses, run number, et cetera.

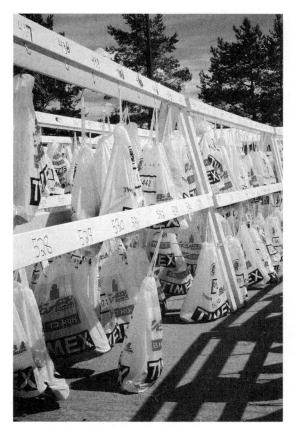

Transition bags at Lake Placid transition area

4. *Two special needs bags—bike and run:*
During long-distance races such as the Ironman, they will often have a place at the halfway points of both the bike and the run where you can pick up a bag that you have filled with any "special needs" you may foresee having at that point. Special nutrition and/or hydration, clothing, anything you feel you may want at mile 56 of the bike and mile 13.1 of the run. You will assemble these bags prior to the race and usually drop them off race morning at special locations.

FAMILIARIZING YOURSELF WITH THE TRIATHLON COURSE

Should you check out the course before your race? Depending on where your triathlon is, this may or may not be an option. Many of you will do triathlons close to home, and you may already train on the course itself or be familiar with the area. Others will see their course for the first time as they race on it. Do you have to study the course and know it inside and out before your race? No. The higher your goals are, then obviously the more familiar you should be with all aspects of the course. You can drive the bike and run the course in your car and take notes, and/or you can ride and run as much as is possible and fits into your training plan if you are shooting for a low finishing time. If your goal is simply to finish, then it is up to you what and how much you wish to find out about the course ahead of the race.

Also, if you are doing a Half-Ironman- or Ironman-distance triathlon, biking the entire course several days before your race is definitely not part of the 12-Week Triathlete training plan. You may feel like you want to do it, but push that feeling aside and taper like you are supposed to.

If it is possible, it is a good idea to get acclimated to the swim course. If all of the buoys and markers are up (they are not always in the water beforehand; some are put out race morning), then getting in the water to determine what you will be sighting off of will help you race morning. Triathlon swims can be configured in many different ways; out and backs, triangles, rectangles, and variations thereof. If the swim is short or several loops and is already marked, then you can swim it beforehand and pick out your landmarks and other potential objects that you can use to guide you during the swim. If you do swim the course beforehand, be sure to swim out and turn around to face the shore, picking the object that you will use to sight off of in your swim to the finish.

You can often find out swim, bike, and run course descriptions on the Web site, in the race literature, and at the prerace meeting. If knowing more about the course and working out on it will help your race, then by all means do it. Being familiar with the course can be more of a mental issue than a physical one, calming your nerves somewhat by making the unknown known. Just make sure that this doesn't cause the opposite effect; some athletes may become more nervous by seeing the course prior to the race and would be better off just racing the course sight unseen. Know yourself and do whatever will help your race, not hurt it.

It is a good idea to "walk" through the entire start of the race, if possible. So, you would go to the swim start, taking a practice swim or just observe the course from shore, then exit from the swim finish and walk the exact line that you will take on race morning to your transition area. By now you should have registered and you know what your race number is; therefore, you can walk to your bike rack spot in transition. Stop and take a good look around, again noticing landmarks to get your bearings. Really make a good mental note of the location of your transition spot. The area may be empty now, but it certainly won't be race morning. Then there will be controlled chaos as you exit the water with any number of other triathletes. You will be slightly lightheaded from your swim, full of adrenaline because you finished the first part of your race, and finding your bike can become a major undertaking if you are not careful. Stand in your bike spot and memorize where you are.

★ KNOW YOUR TRANSITION AREA LOCATION

The Chicago Triathlon is a very popular and very large race, with obviously a huge transition area. There is footage of a race several years ago, and this now-famous transition area; it shows an athlete running up and down the rows of bikes, searching in vain for his transition area. Back and forth, back and forth, and back and forth again. Don't become the prerace entertainment for years to come with your own triathlon blooper; know your transition area location.

SLEEP

The sleep you get two nights before your race is the important night of rest, not the night before. No one really sleeps well that night, and the start times of some races will require that you wake up at 4 or 5 A.M. Try to get as much rest as you can two nights before your race, and do not worry if you stare at the ceiling all night the following night. You are not alone, and it will not affect your race.

THE DAY BEFORE THE RACE

Today you will do the short brick workout. It is not to advance your fitness level at all; this workout serves to keep your legs "fresh," warming up those muscles after your day off and preparing them for tomorrow's race. It is also a last opportunity to make sure that all your gear is in order and your bike is working properly. Use it as a "dress rehearsal," wearing your race clothes for the bike and the run. This last workout will also help to calm your anxiety and release some nervous energy.

When you are done with all of your workouts, it's time to get all of your gear together. If you are competing in a race where you will be setting up your own transition area, then get all of your equipment together and try to choose a bag to carry it all in. I recommend putting on everything that you will wearing one last time and then placing it immediately in this bag. Failure to put things away right away will often lead to items being left out and left behind.

So, stand with all your gear and your registration bag. Put on everything you will be swimming in, from your suit to your cap, goggles, and chip, if your triathlon has provided one. Then, take it all off and place it immediately in this bag, not to be removed until you arrive at your race site.

Do the same with your bike gear. Put your bike outfit on, your helmet, shoes, sunglasses, everything; then take it all off and place it in the bag. Do the same with your run clothing and gear as well.

You may have bike bottles, gel bottles, and Fuel Belt bottles as well. Fill them all now and either place them in a separate plastic bag next to this bag or, if you want them cold, place them in the refrigerator. Do not put them in the same bag as your clothing and gear, as they will most likely leak and possibly explode, and you do not want to find this out race morning. If you do refrigerate them, be sure to put a note on the bag reminding you of this; you will be running around on race morning and it is extremely easy to forget these, and this can be disastrous to your race plans.

You should have already affixed the race numbers to your bike and helmet if provided, before your final short workout.

Bike and Bag Check-In

At some longer-distance races, you will have to check your bike in the day before the race. You will also have to drop off your transition bags as well. This is why it is crucial that you have all the necessary equipment in these bags, and in the correct bags as well! Don't make the mistake of putting your running gear into your bike bag and vice versa—this will really be an unwelcome surprise come race morning!

Yes, there have been stories about triathletes who have made this mistake and ended up biking in their running shoes. I also heard a story about a guy who had started the bike leg of his race and couldn't figure out why the biker in the distance looked so strange, until he got closer and realized that this guy was biking in his wetsuit. I'm guessing he forgot his biking clothes. Don't be this guy.

Most races will now allow you to access these bags on race morning, adding or changing items if you need to. Again, if you can avoid this, do so; it is one less thing to have to worry about on race morning when you will already have many other required things to do. Check with your specific race rules if this is a concern of yours.

One thing that you should be able to bring with you on race morning is your nutrition and hydration. This wasn't always the case. I believe it was Ironman Germany years ago where they insisted you drop everything off the night before and could not get to it before the race; this included all bike bottles, gel bottles, everything. Needless to say, these items were really warm and putrid by the time you used them many hours later. This rule has since been changed, so you can refrigerate your drinks and gels and have fresh bars and whatever other food you choose to bring with you race morning. Just be sure to put them all in one place and remember to bring them with you!

Eating the Day Before

This is definitely not the day to try any new foods. If you have traveled to your race site, do not make the mistake of going out and trying some Indian food or some other new fancy cuisine that you have never tried before. Keep it simple, and stick with what you know. If you have been carbo loading, now's the last chance to get the last few in. Don't overdo it. Don't have a huge meal the night before, which might be too much to handle at 7 the next morning. If you are racing a sprint or Olympic race, this is not as much a concern of yours.

If you are racing the Half-Ironman or Ironman distance and have been taking in additional sodium these last few days, you can continue to do so today. Have some extra pretzels or other salty foods and add a little more salt to your meals.

My race has a carbo dinner—should I go to it?
Some triathlons do have carbo dinners as part of the whole event. They can be a great way to get into the whole spirit of your race and meet some other triathletes. Sometimes this is where the race instructions will be given, and if that is the case, then you should absolutely go. If you do go, don't eat any foods that you have not had before, and don't feel the need to overeat, either. If the carbo dinner is just dinner and not race instructions, and it will make you more nervous or you'd rather eat food you are accustomed to, then by all means do so. If it's your first triathlon and you've never been to a carbo party before, it can be really fun, if for no other reason than to witness the aforementioned Peacock Parade.

So, eat a sensible carbohydrate dinner the night before the race, but don't overdo it. Try to eat early in the evening if possible, to give your body more time to process the food before your swim start.

RACE NUMBERS AND RACE BELTS

Most triathlons will provide you with two race numbers: a bike number and a run number. They often look exactly the same. If you will be changing from your bike jersey to a different run jersey, you can pin the numbers on both jerseys beforehand. The bike number goes on the back of your bike jersey, and the run number goes on the front of your run jersey.

If you do not want to pin the numbers on your clothing or will be biking and running in the same outfit, many athletes choose to use a race belt, a belt that you attach one of these numbers to. For the bike leg, you simply spin it around so that the number is behind you, and for the run you spin it so that the number is on the front.

Again, be very careful to check the rules to make sure that there are no special policies governing your race. As I discussed earlier with my experience in Australia, sometimes race organizers will have rules that vary from the normal way of doing things, such as having to use both race numbers. To deal with this situation and still use a race belt, I attached both numbers onto my race belt with the bike number on top. When I finished the bike leg, I spun the number back around and ripped it off, leaving on the run number.

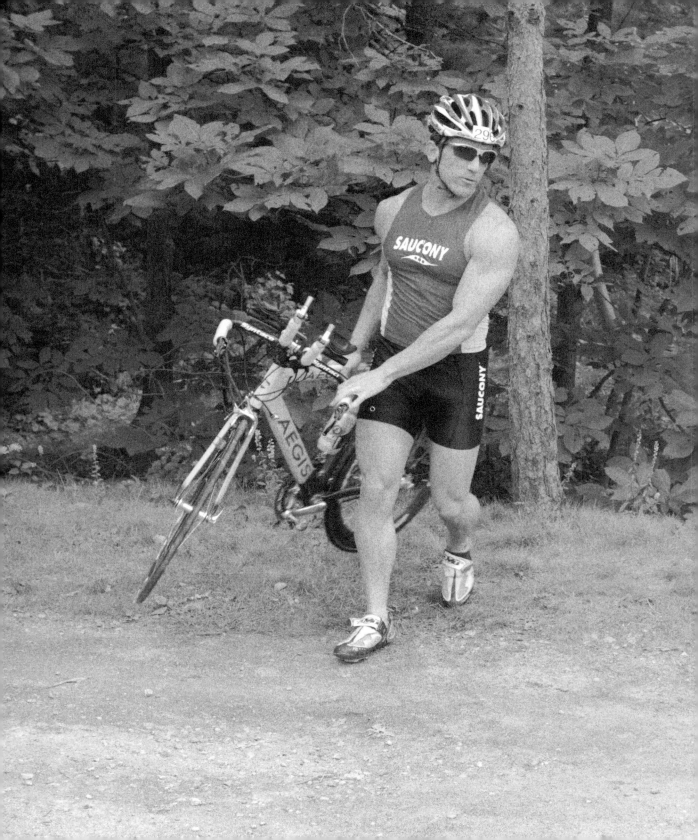

CHAPTER 13
Race Day

WAKE-UP TIME

Most of you will probably be smart and give yourself plenty of time to get ready in the morning, but this point bears repeating. Don't plan on waking up a half hour before your race—there are many things you will need to do and you do not want to be running around and wasting valuable energy. I would generally plan on getting up at least two hours before race start to adequately prepare yourself. You will need to eat, use the bathroom, set up your transition area or check on your bike, use the bathroom, get bodymarked, use the bathroom, and yes, inevitably something will go wrong and you will need extra time to deal with it. And then you will need to use the bathroom again. It is better to have extra time to warm up and stretch than to cut it too close and start your race stressed out or even late, for that matter.

THE WEATHER

I check the weather report before a race only to see if I need to wear something different, and even then the weather rarely changes anything. I might add arm warmers if it will be cold at the beginning of the bike, but that's usually the extent of the changes. Do not make the mistake of obsessing about the weather. Hopefully you trained in almost all possible conditions—heat, cold, wind, rain, as well as on beautiful days.

There are two important points you should realize about the weather:

1. You can't control it.
2. Everyone in the race will be experiencing the same exact weather as you will.

Let me repeat that point because I believe it is an essential mental aspect of racing—everyone will be experiencing the same conditions that you will on race day, so don't feel sorry for yourself! It will only lessen your race performance and enjoyment. This also holds true with the race course—everyone will swim in the same cold water, bike and run up the same hills, big and small, to get to that finish line.

If they can do it, so can you.

THE RACE

Game day.

Here's where the fun begins!

You can't believe the day is now here. It seems like only yesterday that you made the decision to sign up for this race. You've trained consistently and adhered to workouts in all three disciplines, you did your strength training, and you stretched as well. Hopefully you tried some visualization and relaxation exercises, too. The hard physical work has ended, and now it's game day! If you have worked hard and are injury-free, then congratulations! You are in the minority and should be really proud of yourself. I tell all my clients that my primary job and goal as a coach is to get them to that start line without any major injuries. I cannot tell you how many people start their races injured, and it does not have to be that way. Of course you may be sore. You may have some small aches and pains and tight muscles as well. That's normal! Given all the training you have done, this is to be expected. And remember that the mind does some funny things as we get really close to our race. Suddenly everything hurts, and we seem to hurt ourselves sleeping and just lying around.

All of these aches and pains and doubts will be erased the moment that starter's pistol goes off. Adrenaline is our body's own natural wonder drug.

At some point on this day, really stop for a moment and take pride in what you have done and what you are about to do. It may sound corny, but you have done great things for your body and your mind. You have invested in your health, you have set goals for yourself, and you are about to challenge yourself. The race is now just the final party to celebrate all of your hard work and dedication.

Race Morning

Maybe you slept well, most likely you didn't. You may have fallen asleep but had a gut-wrenching TSD where something went horribly wrong with your race. The great thing about these dreams is waking up from them and realizing that it didn't actually happen! Your stomach may be in knots now; your heart rate may be slowly inching up into your Race Pace zone already.

Yet again, normal. Relax.

If you feel great, that's great! If you don't feel great, tell yourself that you do. It is now time to begin your self-talk statements, whatever works for you. From the moment you open your eyes, you should fill your head with these statements:

"I feel great."

"Today's my day."

"I feel strong."

Goofy? Maybe. Effective? Absolutely. Are the elite athletes doing the same thing? Absolutely. No doubt about it.

Bathroom

Now this is not a topic that I am particularly fond of talking or writing about, but unfortunately it is a crucial aspect of your prerace preparations. You need to go to the bathroom, and you need to go to the bathroom frequently. And no matter how many times you go to the bathroom before your race, yes, you will still have to go one more time seconds before the gun goes off.

So, the minute you wake up, use the bathroom. Then you should eat your breakfast to give your body time to digest before the swim start.

Race Morning Breakfast

By now you should really have a good idea about what you should eat for breakfast—it's whatever has been working for you before your longer workouts. Like dinner the night before, this is not a time to try something new; stick with what you know. You do want to eat something, as your energy stores were slightly depleted as you slept. A breakfast that you are used to that contains carbohydrates is what you should eat. The longer your triathlon, the more important this breakfast can be to your performance, so try not to skip this meal.

If you are traveling to your race, prepare ahead and bring your breakfast with you if possible. You will not always be able to find your specific foods when you travel, and if you must have this breakfast, take it along.

Last-Minute Preparations

Next, get dressed in your swim outfit, and if the race will be using chip timing, be sure to put that on now as well. For triathlon, the chip is most often secured to your ankle with a strip of Velcro. Put it on immediately. You may also want to wear sweats and a long-sleeve shirt to keep you warm until race start. Even in summer the mornings can be cold, and you don't want to be walking around shivering.

Now use the bathroom one more time before you leave.

So, it's time to go. Grab your bag with all of your gear, grab your nutrition and hydration items that you may have refrigerated, and grab your bike.

Should I bring my floor bike pump with me?

You will want to inflate your tires one last time in the transition area, so you will need a floor pump to effectively do this. You can bring your own or do as many other triathletes do and simply borrow one from somebody else in the transition area. There will inevitably be someone close to your transition spot who will have brought a pump that you can use. If you do bring your own pump, be prepared to lend it out yourself.

ARRIVING AT THE RACE

You arrive at the race site. Most likely you are really nervous now. It is probably still dark, but through the darkness you see the outlines of all these fancy bikes and triathletes who all have the bodies and outfits of professionals. The majority of them are thinking and feeling the exact same way you are.

Bodymarking

You will usually have to be bodymarked before being allowed to enter the transition area. At the bodymarking stations, a volunteer will write your race numbers on your body with a pen; usually on one or both of your shoulders and your thighs, and often your age or a letter that indicates your age group will be written on your calf as well. Thank the volunteer and continue on to your transition area.

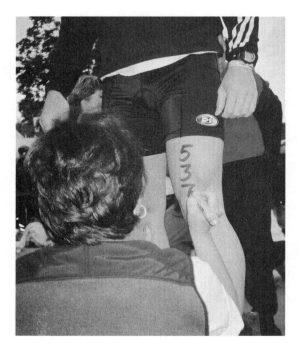

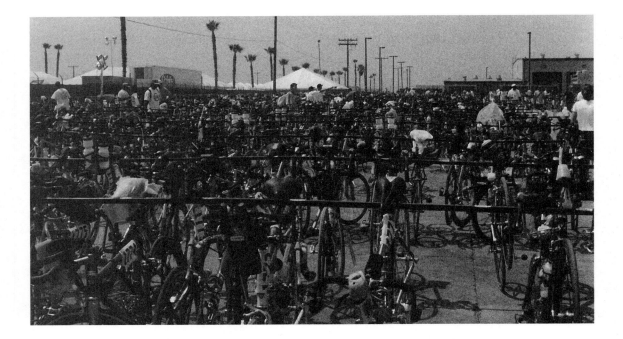

If you will be using sunscreen, and I highly recommend you do, unless your triathlon takes place indoors, do not put it on before being bodymarked, as it forms a perfect protective shield against the ink of the marker. Apply your sunscreen right after being bodymarked, and when you do, be careful when spreading it over your newly numbered areas, as it also serves as a perfect ink removal solution.

TRANSITION AREA

For those of you who have no idea what the transition area is, it is merely an area filled with rows of numbered bike racks. They may be 1 through 50, 50 through 100, and so on. You simply find your number on the rack, and that is where your bike is to go. For the smaller races, this is also where all your gear will go, in a spot right next to your bike. For those doing bigger triathlons that involve changing tents and transition bags, your bike is the only thing that goes here, except maybe your bike shoes attached to your pedals.

This is one of the areas where different races have different rules. For those races where you will not be setting up a transition area, some allow only your bike in this spot and that's it; others may allow you to attach your bike shoes. Check your race packet if this is a concern of yours.

If you are doing a longer-distance triathlon such as the Ironman that entails using transition bags, then most likely you dropped off your bike and bags the night before. You do not need to set up your transition, but you still have a few things to attend to.

1. Put your all the hydration and nutrition that you will be using on your bike.
2. Make sure that your tires are properly inflated.

I say "properly inflated" because one of the common sounds in the transition area is the loud report of bike tires exploding from overinflation. Do not let your nerves get the best of you and put too much air in your tires—changing a flat race morning is not a great way to start the day. And just because the tires do not pop right before the race, many that have been overinflated will actually pop while you are swimming as the day heats up and the air in the tires expands. You certainly do not want to come out from the swim and find one or both of your tires flat—properly inflate them.

Many triathlons will have a local bike shop at the transition area that will be able to help you with any last-minute bike emergencies. Be aware that these people will be scrambling to help many triathletes in distress, and you may have to wait for their assistance. If something does go wrong with your bike and you cannot fix it, do not wait, seek them out immediately. Ask another triathlete for help only as a last resort, as he or she has his or her own prerace preparations to attend to and may not have any time to spare.

Make sure that your bike is in a small (low equals easy) gear as well before you put it on the rack. You don't want to jump on the bike pumped full of adrenaline from just having completed the swim and then topple over on the bike because the gear was too big. Many races will even add insult to injury by starting immediately on a steep uphill—if you get on your bike in too big a gear, you may not make it up your first climb.

For those of you that will be setting up your entire transition area, you will need to lay out all of your gear in the small area provided to

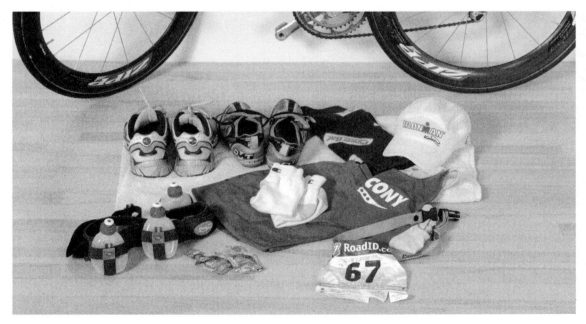

A mock transition area

you. This is why it is a good idea to get to the transition area as soon as possible—you want to "claim your space" before all of the triathletes around you have claimed theirs, and perhaps more than theirs. There should be adequate room for everyone to set up their gear. You only need a small rectangular-shaped area on either side of your bike to place all of your gear.

The following is a list you can follow when setting up your transition area. You may have more or fewer items and much of this will come down to personal preference over time, but this is a general outline you can follow when setting up your area:

1. *Place your bike on the rack.* You can do this by hooking either the handlebars or the seat on the rack, whichever you prefer.

Some race directors like all the bikes to be racked either frontward or backward, so if everyone else's bike is racked a certain way, you should probably follow their lead and place yours the same way. Remember to make sure that the bike is in an easy gear to start your ride.

2. *Pick a spot either to the right or left of your bike—this is where you will place your gear.* I recommend placing a towel down in this spot, generally a large towel folded in half. This is now your area.

3. *Put on your helmet and buckle it to make sure it works.* Things as simple as a chin strap can break without your knowing it, and without it fastened, you cannot race.

4. *Place all your gear on this towel.* Helmet, bike shoes, running shoes, any

---

⭐ **SLOW AND STEADY**

If your goal is simply to finish your triathlon, I highly recommend that you slow down as much as possible during your transitions and take your time. So many people sprint through these transitions, and they would do much better if they just took a few extra moments. By trying to save a few precious seconds here, they end up not doing something like putting on antichafing gel or sunscreen or putting on their sunglasses or the bandana they are accustomed to wearing, and they end up paying for it later. Many triathletes also slip and fall while in transition, some seriously, while putting on their gear or trying to mount their bikes and ride off immediately. So, take your time. Take a few deep breaths. Do everything you planned on doing and practiced doing. Taking thirty extra seconds in transition can really pay off later in the race, especially for those of you who will be doing longer-distance triathlons.

clothing you will be changing into, sunglasses, a towel to dry off with, et cetera. Place them in a systematic way so that it will be easy for you to grab them when the time comes, when there will be people rushing all around you and you will feel rushed as well. You should have practiced this at least once in your training and thus have some idea how you want to arrange your gear.

5. Take your bike back off the rack and inflate your tires. Remember to not overdo it.
6. Rerack your bike.
7. Mentally go through your gear one final time visually to ensure that you have all your gear in place.
8. Leave.

I say "leave" because I have watched many nervous triathletes spend too much time in the transition area. They fiddle with this and fiddle with that, often resulting in their screwing something up that was otherwise perfectly fine. Your bike should have been tuned-up already, so you should have nothing much to do except inflate your tires and put down your gear.

My triathlon will have a beach swim and then we will run on the sand to the transition area. Won't my feet be covered with sand? What's the best way to clean them off before I put on my bike shoes?

You can use your extra towel at your transition area to dry off as well as clean off your feet. The easiest way to get the sand off of your feet is to sit on your transition spot and wipe your feet clean—trying to do it while standing can be a little difficult and not very effective.

You can also bring a small pail or large plastic container of water and leave it at your transition area. You simply step in it to get the sand off of your feet and then towel them dry.

What about changing clothes? I want to change from my wet bathing suit into dry bike shorts; how do I do this if they don't have a changing tent?

Use your extra towel to cover yourself after you dry off. Wrap it around yourself, remove the wetsuit, and pull on your dry clothes. Although many people seem to lose all inhibitions about public nudity in transition areas, try to cover up when changing. Some race directors will penalize or disqualify you if you choose to give a free peep show at your transition area.

THE SWIM

Now you need to prepare yourself for the swim. Begin by using the restroom one more time. If you are like many triathletes, you have some apprehension about this part of the race. Take a few extra deep breaths and continue to engage in your positive self-talk statements. This is when they really make a difference.

Next, you will want to put on sunscreen, one that is waterproof and with a high SPF. Choosing not to put on sunscreen can be a big mistake and can actually affect your race performance. Having sunburned skin will negatively affect your body's cooling system, not a good thing during a hot race.

If you are swimming without a wetsuit, then all you will really need are your goggles, your swim cap, which they most likely have provided, a timing chip if the race will be timed

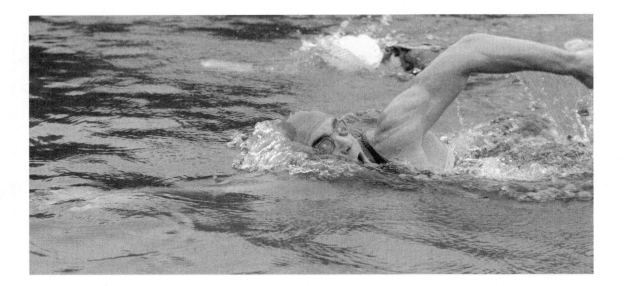

this way, and your swim suit, which you ideally are already wearing.

If you will be wearing a wetsuit, then you want to start putting it on at least fifteen minutes before the race start to give yourself enough time to get it on properly and just in case you have any unforeseen issues. Don't wait until the last minute to put it on; you never know what might happen. Of course, you will want to put on your sunscreen before you begin to deal with your wetsuit.

Wetsuits can be difficult to get on, and there are a couple of simple ways to make this process easier.

1. *Plastic bags:* You put plastic bags over both feet as you pull up the wetsuit, to allow it to slide up easier and not get stuck to your skin. You do the same with your upper body, putting the bags on your hands as you pull your arms through the sleeves.

2. *Body Glide:* You rub a product like Body Glide on your body parts that get stuck on the wetsuit as you pull it on. This should also help you when pulling it off. Some triathletes have taken to using the home cooking spray Pam as a lubricant, spraying it on their bodies to minimize this friction.

One note about the wetsuits; if you are wearing one that has a long string attached to the zipper, you want to fold the string in two and place the folded end under the Velcro strap at the back of your neck. This is to prevent some major chafing issues; if you leave this long piece of string out, it can rub on your neck and leave a nasty burn at the end of your swim as a result. I failed to do this before a long Ironman swim, and it looked like I had tried to hang myself when I emerged from the water 2.4 miles later. Even when you fold this string over it can still rub; I recommend putting some lubricant such as Body Glide on the back of your neck to avoid any chafing issues.

Can't I just use good old Vaseline to avoid chafing issues and make putting on my wetsuit and taking it off easier?

No. Wetsuits are made of neoprene and Vaseline will eat away at this material.

If you will be using both a timing chip and a wetsuit, be sure that the timing ship is under your wetsuit and not over it. It should be attached to your ankle and be under the suit or just below it if your wetsuit legs sit above your ankles. If you attach this chip over your suit, then it will come off when you remove your wetsuit—not something you want to have happen. You will have a time logged for the swim and no record of your finishing the bike or the run.

Allrighty then. Your transition area is all set up; your swim outfit is on. You have applied your sunscreen, you have your goggles and swim cap, and if they gave you one, you have your timing chip on as well. You are ready to race.

Some triathletes like to get in the water a little early and swim around a little bit to loosen up. Others prefer to stretch on shore and enter the water at race start. Whatever you choose as your prerace ritual, just make sure to do something to get your blood flowing and your muscles loosened up. Jogging in place, an easy out-and-back swim, shoulder stretches, and so on. Take a final look out at the swim course and make mental notes of the buoys and what you will be sighting off of. When there are just a few minutes until your race start, put on your swim cap and adjust your goggles. Take a few more deep breaths and start thinking of your most positive self-talk statements. Put a big smile on your face, get your watch ready if you plan on timing yourself, and wait for that starter's gun or horn to break through the morning air.…

The Swim Start

Once again, your swim may take place in staggered wave starts or you may all go together in a mass wave start. Whatever the case, you have to decide whether or not you want to get right in the middle of it all and swim with the masses or avoid the bodies and the chaos and swim with a little more room.

★ **BE CAREFUL WITH PAM**

This may sound like fiction, but it's true—be sure to pay close attention to what you are buying if you choose to use the Pam method. More than one triathlete has sprayed this product on themselves in transition only to realize that they have just coated themselves with Pam with garlic—and are forced to race smelling like the kitchen of an Italian restaurant.

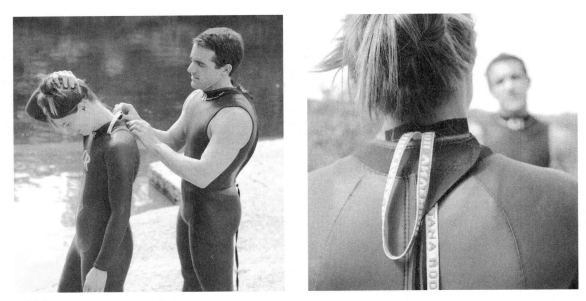

Fold zipper strap to prevent chafing

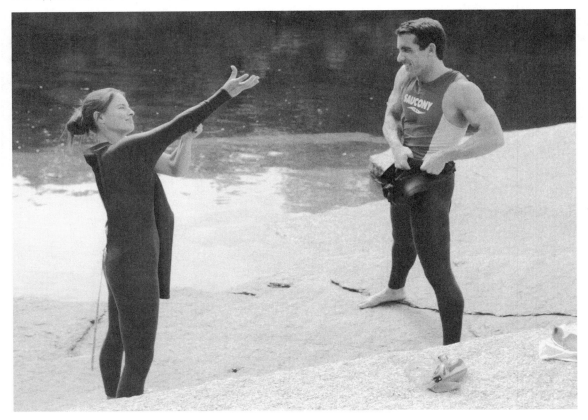

ESCAPE FROM ALCATRAZ

The Escape from Alcatraz is an incredible race and one that I recommend highly. There are currently two versions of this race, and both are beautiful triathlons of approximately Olympic distances. When I participated in it, we boarded two barges that were to take us out to the island (you begin the swim by jumping off of these boats at the shore rather than starting on the shore itself). During the trip out to Alcatraz, I struck up a conversation with a fellow triathlete, and we discussed our past race experiences. As the start time grew close, I began to put on my wetsuit and noticed that he was making no attempt to put on his. When I reminded him how close we were to the race start, he remarked that he had plenty of time to get ready. As I zippered up my suit and we were but minutes from taking the icy plunge, he slowly began to pull on his suit. When he went to zipper his up with about a minute to spare, he reached back and pulled at the zipper, which broke off in his hand. He looked at me with terror in his eyes and asked me to fix it for him. I fumbled with it for a few moments and was unsuccessful in trying to put it back on. As we were but thirty seconds from the swim start, I handed it back to him and apologized for not being able to help. He now had about ten seconds to decide what to do—to swim without it (these waters are frigid, just above fifty degrees), swim with it on and open in the back, or not swim at all. These are not decisions you want to be making just before your triathlon start, especially a swim as challenging as the one from Alcatraz to shore. Give yourself plenty of time to prepare for your swim. (For those of you who are wondering, he ended up jumping in with the wetsuit wide open in the back—although I never saw him again, I assume he finished the swim, but I cannot imagine that it was a comfortable one given his damaged wetsuit dragging him down and letting in that icy cold water.)

If you are like many triathletes and the thought of swimming in a big group doesn't particularly appeal to you, then you have a few ways to avoid this.

1. When the gun goes off to start, count slowly to ten or so, letting the stronger swimmers and the loonies go first; then slowly enter the water and begin your swim.

2. Start "outside." In other words, start a little outside of the group and make your way back toward the inside as you swim. For instance, if you will be swimming straight out and turning right at the final buoy, then start your swim more to the left of the main group. You will then swim at a diagonal toward that final buoy while avoiding swimming with the masses. You will indeed swim a little farther as a result, but this can be a small price to pay to avoid the stress and physical contact that can come from swimming with the main group.

3. If you are really apprehensive about the swim, do both! Count to ten and swim on

the outside to ensure that you will be swimming in your own space. If you are really, really apprehensive, then count to thirty and start even farther outside.

If you do choose to swim with the main group, then just be prepared for some physical contact. There will be punching and kicking as the triathletes jockey for swim space and settle into their swim rhythms. Depending on the size of the area that you will be swimming in, this chaos may or may not subside as the swim progresses. Small-lake swims can be much more chaotic for much longer than, say, an ocean swim, as there is never really any space to spread out into. "Seed" yourself accordingly if you plan to start in the middle of things; in other words, if you are not a particularly strong or fast swimmer, then it is not a good idea to start right at the front. You will be punched and kicked and people will swim right over you if you start too far in front.

Wherever you start, remember that a triathlon consists of three different parts; don't spend all of your energy on the swim. Relax and swim at your own pace. You most likely will get jostled around wherever you choose to start; don't let it rattle you. Remind yourself that every single person around you is experiencing the same thing. If they can handle it, you can handle it. Yes, every race does have athletes who need to be pulled from the water due to panic attacks. You may experience moments of panic yourself during the swim. Your heart rate will suddenly take off and you may experience real feelings of fear. You can slow down, switch to breaststroke, even tread water for a while if you have to. It is actually not against the rules to hang on to a buoy or even to a volunteer in a canoe or on a surfboard if you have to, as long as they are not moving forward. Just get some good breaths of air and call upon both your relaxation and self-talk exercises, which you ideally have practiced during your training. This is exactly the time when you should use them and when they are extremely effective in calming your fears.

Drafting During the Swim

Once again, while drafting may be illegal during the bike portion of your triathlon, it is not during the swim, and if you can do it, you should. As you begin the swim, try following behind different people until you find someone who is swimming at your pace. Try to stay right on his or her toes without hitting him or her. Watch his or her trail of bubbles under the water and follow that as much as possible, rather than lifting your head to sight. You do want to lift your head and look several times as you start to follow this person, just to make sure he or she is traveling in a straight line and not taking you way off course. Once you feel comfortable that this person indeed has a good sense of direction, then you can just settle into a rhythm and follow the underwater trail.

If this person speeds up or slows down too much, then you need to slide away from him or her and continue at your own pace. Try to find another person swimming at your speed and begin to follow him or her. You might draft behind one person the entire swim, or you might have to switch between three or four different swimmers before the swim leg is completed.

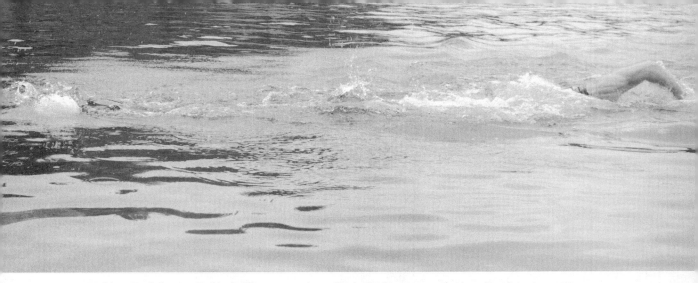

Drafting: Try following behind different people until you find someone who is swimming at your pace

Exiting the Swim

Before you know it you will have finished the swim. Congratulations! You may have swum your desired time, you may have been faster, or you may have been significantly slower. Whatever the case, hit the lap button on your watch if you are timing each leg and then shift your attention to the next leg of the triathlon. Do not focus too heavily on your swim time because it can be affected by many outside factors.

I participated in the now defunct Ironman California years ago, which took place on the marine base Camp Pendleton. The marines were incredible hosts; lining the course and serving as volunteers at the aid stations—it was a truly incredible experience. There was one small problem with the swim, however. When I exited the swim and checked my watch, I was shocked to see a significantly slower time than I usually swim. I immediately began beating myself up mentally, and it took quite some time before I was able to let go of the negative emotions from

having swum so slowly. Well, come to find out several days after the race, that they had, in fact, mismeasured the swim course long. This was such a great lesson in not being attached to swimming a specific time—everyone had swum this same long course and therefore we all had slower times than normal. So, if you really let it affect you or even give up as a result, you are doing yourself an incredible disservice. It is perfectly fine to expect finish times for all three legs of your triathlon, but there are many things that can affect these times, one example being race director error. Other factors can include tides, wind, heat, and the layout of the course—all impact your times. Sure, you might be slower, but everyone else will be as well. Race your race and don't be attached to your watch.

As you exit the water, if you are wearing a wetsuit, you can pull it down around your waist. Remove your swim cap and goggles and jog or run in a controlled manner to your transition spot.

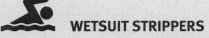

WETSUIT STRIPPERS

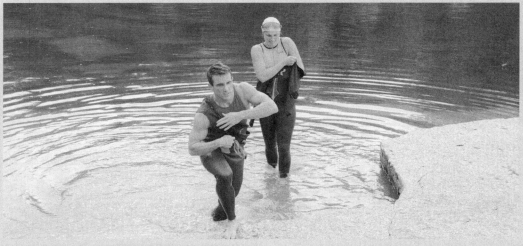

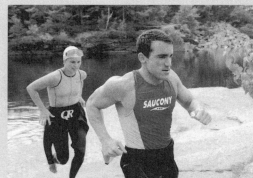

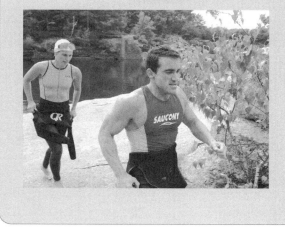

At some of the bigger Half-Ironman- and Ironman-distance races, they will have volunteer wetsuit strippers. The sole job of these people is to pull your wetsuit off of you. As you exit the water, they will be motioning for you to come to them. Have your wetsuit down around your waist as you jog over to them and immediately drop onto your butt in front of one of these volunteers. Lift your legs and lean back; this person will then pull your wetsuit off of you in one motion. You then stand, thank the volunteer for his or her help, and jog on to your transition area or changing tent.

TRANSITION ONE (T1):
THE SWIM-TO-BIKE TRANSITION

If you are participating in a race where you set up your own transition area, then jog over to it and begin to change into your bike gear. Yes, it is a race, and you may have set a lofty time goal for yourself, but remember to take your time to ensure you do everything you need to do and do it correctly. There will most likely be mass chaos going on around you; try not to get caught up in it. Put on blinders and focus on yourself and what you need to do. Ignore everything else going on around you. Dry yourself off, wipe you feet clean, and put on all of your gear. You can reapply sunscreen now as well as some more antichafing product if you wish. Make sure that you put on your helmet and fasten your chinstrap before even taking your bike off of the rack. Exiting this transition area without having your chinstrap fastened is grounds for immediate disqualification in most races. When you are sure that you have everything you need, unrack your bike and begin to walk slowly to the bike exit. Most races will have a designated point where you will be allowed to mount your bike; don't try to ride it before this point or you may be issued a penalty or disqualified. When you get to this point, take a look around you quickly to make sure that you have room to get on your bike—many adrenaline-filled triathletes will often crash into one another at this point as they scramble to take off on their bikes. If the coast is clear, mount your bike and exit T1. One leg down, two to go!

For those of you who will be racing triathlons that involve using transition bags and changing tents, this process will be slightly different. Once you have exited the swim, and your wetsuit, if you wore one, is off, you will begin to jog toward the rows of bags filled with all the triathletes' swim-to-bike gear. Although you should have walked through this the day before to practice your specific route, you will most likely have volunteers who will see your number on you and direct you to your row. You can also call out your number as you approach them so that they can guide you in the appropriate direction as quickly as possible. You will then jog to your bag, grab it, then take it into the changing tent. Depending on how your swim went, this area or tent may be empty or filled with other triathletes and volunteers. If there is a free chair, grab it; if not, try to find an empty area and drop onto your butt. These volunteers are there to help you make this transition and will help you with whatever you need. If you don't need their help, then simply thank them and tell them you are okay on your own. If you do need assistance, then tell them what you need and they will help you out. Remember that they are indeed volunteering their time and be courteous to them at all times. You will dump out the contents of your bag and then put back in your wetsuit, goggles, cap, and any other clothing or items that you will be taking off. Take your time and put on all your bike gear. You can leave the bag with all of your swim gear in the tent, as it has your number on it and will be waiting for you with all your other bags at the race finish. Fasten your chinstrap on your helmet before exiting the transition area, thank the volunteers, and follow the other triathletes and the directions of the volunteers toward your bike.

In these bigger races, you may also have volunteers in T1 who will put sunscreen on

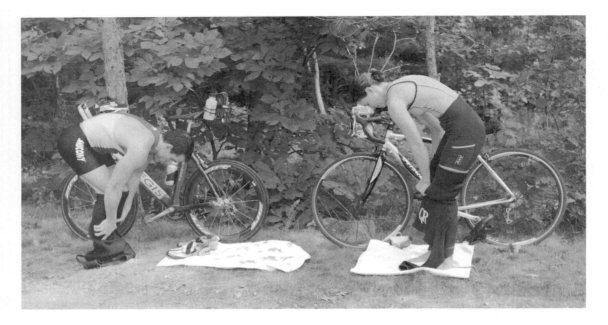

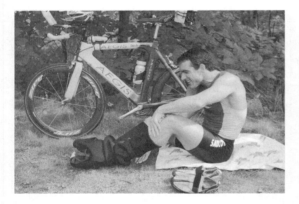

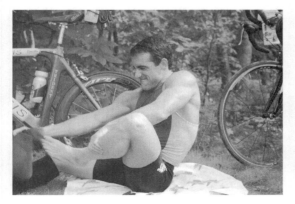

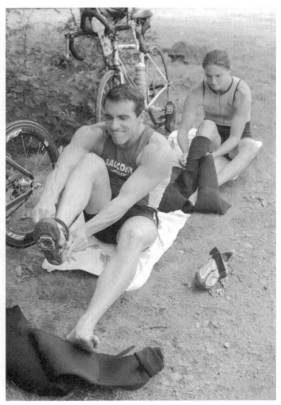

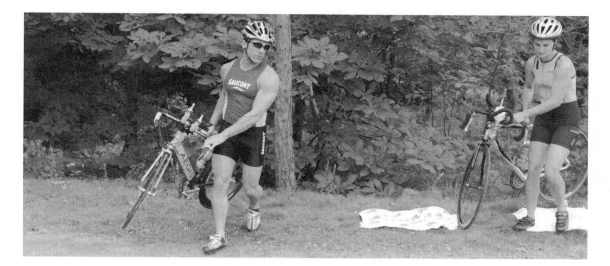

you if you wish, and volunteers who will be offering you Vaseline to put on those areas prone to chafing. If you think you need these things, take advantage of them—don't pass these people by simply to save a few seconds, as you will pay the price later.

There may also be Porta Potties in T1. I know it may seem unfathomable that you have to go again given the half-dozen times you went before the race, but chances are you will. Take the time and use the bathroom rather than be uncomfortable during the entire bike ride. If you haven't discovered this already, it's really difficult to ride in the aero position with a full bladder.

So, you now will run through the rows of bikes toward yours. Once again, the volunteers will be trying to assist you by looking at your number and guiding you to your area. You can call out your number and may even have your bike unracked and waiting for you at the end of your row.

Don't expect the volunteers to do everything for you in transition. They are there to help out as much as possible, but they all have a tough job to do. Call out your number when you can and follow their directions. They may have twenty triathletes asking them for help at the same time and obviously cannot assist everyone at once. This is why it is so helpful to have walked through your race transitions prior to the race—you should really already know where to go and any help from volunteers is extremely helpful but not to be expected.

Take your bike, walk it to the designated mounting spot, get on, and off you go.

Many slower-swimming triathletes, especially first-timers, get down on themselves when they finish the swim and see how few bikes are left in the transition area, how many people are now ahead of them. If you find yourself in this situation, put it out of your mind and remind yourself that triathlon consists of three parts, the shortest of which is the swim. It's not who goes the fastest, it's who slows down the least. Take this as a challenge and see how many triathletes you can "reel in," slowly passing on both the bike and the run.

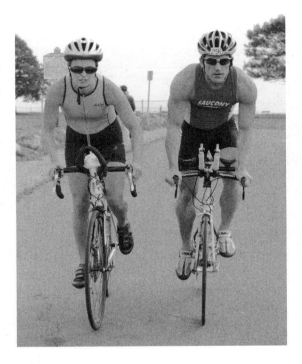

as much as possible while holding your pace. If you are doing a long-distance triathlon, then every twenty minutes or so do a few quick stretches to stay loose and prevent any cramping. This is especially important if you will be riding in the aero position for much of the bike leg. Twist your shoulders to one side and then to the other while sitting up to stretch your back muscles. Stand occasionally and arch your back to stretch it out as well. Do whatever you need to do to remain relaxed, and do it before you feel soreness rather than when it is too late. Just like your nutrition, stretch and relax your body at regular intervals.

Nutrition and Hydration

By your race you should know almost exactly what your nutrition and hydration strategy will be. You have practiced it numerous times during your workouts, especially your longer ones. You have figured out what works for you and what does not. Do not change anything on race day unless you have absolutely no choice.

Once again, you want to try to get in at least twenty ounces of liquid per hour on the bike and approximately 250 to 400 calories as well. Drink and eat at regular intervals, roughly every ten to fifteen minutes or so, depending on what you have become accustomed to.

Some believe you should wait ten minutes or so after your swim to eat or drink anything, until you have settled down from the swim. I don't necessarily believe this to be a rule set in stone and personally have no issues with taking in a little nutrition and fluids soon into the bike leg. Again, do what works for you.

For those of you doing longer-distance triathlons, it has been my experience that feeling

THE BIKE LEG

So, you have finished the swim, successfully navigated through T1, and are now off on the bike leg. Take a moment to congratulate yourself for completing the swim and then shift your focus to the task at hand.

Like in any other race, many people will start out way too fast. This holds true with the swim start of the triathlon and with the bike start as well. Do not fall into the trap of trying to hammer along with the majority of triathletes who are going out too fast at the beginning of the bike. Many of these athletes will suffer the consequences of going out too hard, and if you stick to your pace, you will inevitably pass many of them on the run course.

Stay relaxed on the bike. Constantly do body checks from head to toe and see if you are holding tension anywhere. Relax all your muscles a little queasy while following your eating and drinking schedule can be normal. In other words, do not immediately take this feeling as a sign that you need to pull back from your timetable. What you need to realize is that being dehydrated or running low on energy will be a lot worse later on than a mildly upset stomach. Some people seem to have stronger stomachs than others do and can tolerate more discomfort from eating and drinking while exercising. This is truly where individual toughness and knowledge of one's own body come into play. Also realize that this part of your racing is never truly perfected and outside factors will affect it from race to race. Professional triathletes are constantly tweaking their nutrition and hydration strategies and often drop out of races due to gastrointestinal upset. So, no matter how much you practice all this during your training, it will always change slightly on race day. This is yet another never-ending learning process. If the pros can have issues with their nutrition and hydration, then you certainly can also. The body does not really like taking in food and drink when exercising at high intensities, yet it needs both of these to perform, so trouble is inevitable and can only be controlled rather than cured.

Just to give you some idea of what a nutrition and hydration strategy might look like on the bike, the following is an outline of my current Ironman plan. It, too, is forever undergoing little changes and modifications as I learn more through each workout and every race.

Carried on the bike to start:
1. One 28-ounce bike bottle filled with Ensure: 1,050 calories
2. One 20-ounce bike bottle filled with Gatorade: 125 calories
3. One PowerGel flask filled with 3 PowerGels and water: 300 calories

At the aid stations:
4. Alternating between drinking one 20-ounce bottle of Gatorade or the equivalent and one 20-ounce bottle of water every hour
5. One energy bar (200 calories) and one banana (100 calories)

Over the course of roughly a 5-and-a-half-hour bike leg, I would then take in just over 2,000 calories, or 400 calories per hour. This is a little on the high end, but I have found that I do not perform well taking in fewer calories. As you can see, the majority of the calories are in liquid form, with a small percentage of the total calories coming from solid and semisolid form.

Aid Stations

During your triathlon, you will most likely have at least one aid station on the bike course and many more for longer races. It is here that you will take additional nutrition and liquids from the volunteers who are manning each location. There is a certain technique involved in this exchange. As you approach the aid station, begin to slow down. Make sure that there is no one directly in front of you or directly behind you as you slow down, as accidents are common at the aid stations. That rider in front of you may come to a screeching halt and you will crash into him or her, or that person behind you will be looking at the volunteers and not notice that you have slowed down, potentially hitting you from behind. Once the

BIKE BOTTLES: NO RETURN

If your water bottles have some significance to you, then you should not bring them to the race—most likely you will not be able to retrieve them afterward. Whatever bottles you end up with at the end of the race are now yours, and yours are now theirs. So, if you absolutely love the race bottle you got at your last race, leave it at home and bring generic ones to the race.

coast is clear and you have slowed down, you should approach the aid station with the following in mind:

1. If you need to get rid of any water bottles that you have finished and replace them, you will throw them just before the aid station itself. Many stations will have a clearly marked area where you are to aim and "jettison" your empty bottles.

2. As you pass through the aid station, the volunteers will be holding water bottles and other items out with arms extended. You simply reach out and take it from them with soft hands, thank the volunteer, place it on your bike, and pick up your pace again. You may need to take more than one item from each station, so make sure that you slow down enough to give yourself time to get everything you need.

3. At the bigger races, they may have six or more items to choose from at the aid stations, including water, Gatorade, energy bars, PowerGels, and bananas. As you approach the station, the volunteers will be calling out what they each have to offer, and you can begin to call out what you need as well. You will then see a volunteer who has what you need move toward

you; make eye contact with him or her and then take it.

Your body needs fluids to function properly. Don't skip these aid stations, and stick to the drinking plan that you have practiced during your workouts. Don't wait until the later aid stations to get your fluids, either; you need to drink throughout the entire bike course. Remember that, once you are thirsty, it's too late—you're already dehydrated.

What do I have to do if I need to go to the bathroom while I'm on the bike?

Some larger triathlons will have Porta Potties on the bike and run courses, but this is rare for most races. You have essentially two options in this department:

1. Find an appropriate place on the side of the road and be discreet.

2. Just go. Yes, without stopping—just go.

Obviously, the second option is reserved for those who truly have a performance goal in mind. Going while on the bike is a skill in and of itself and also requires some practice. This is all I will say on this subject; you choose whichever option you wish to exercise. Just be nice and warn riders behind you if and when you choose option number 2.

Just to hammer these two points home one more time, here are the two main things you need to remember about the bike leg of your triathlon:

1. You will have to run afterward and will pay the price if you bike too hard. I would argue that, for every minute you go too hard on the bike, your run time will suffer several minutes or more.

2. You want to get the majority of your calories and fluids in while on the bike. Your body will not be as accepting of these two things while you are running.

The bike sets up the run. Remember that point and you will have a great race.

TRANSITION TWO (T2): THE BIKE-TO-RUN TRANSITION

As you approach your transition area at the end of the bike leg, there is most often a "dismount line." Similar to the bike mount line at T1, this is the place where you must get off of your bike and then walk your bike back to your transition area. Most times, there will be volunteers calling out for you to slow down before this point and then calling out for you to stop before this line. Make sure you follow their directions. Failure to get off your bike at this point can result in penalties or disqualification. It is for your own safety and the safety of your fellow triathletes.

If you have set up your own transition area, then you will walk your bike back to your spot and change into your run gear. Unless you have a serious time goal set for yourself at a shorter-distance triathlon, take your time and don't run. Many triathletes try to sprint back to their transition area and end up falling or crashing into other people as a result. Bike shoes can be very difficult to run in and you can easily lose your footing while running in them.

Once you arrive at your spot, you will rerack your bike and begin to change into your run gear. You can take this opportunity to take in some additional calories and fluids if you need to. Take your time and do everything you planned on doing. There will be a run exit out of the transition, where you will begin the final leg of your triathlon.

For those of you doing the longer-distance races, the drill is the same with transition bags

BIKE CATCHERS

At some Half-Ironman- and Ironman-distance races, there are volunteers who are known as "bike catchers." After you dismount your bike, these volunteers will take your bike from you, take it back to your spot on the bike rack, and rerack it for you.

as for T1. You will enter T2, get rid of your bike, and then pick up your bike-to-run bag. These bags will often be lined up in rows, and you will be guided toward your bag by the volunteers. You can call out your number and make sure your race number is visible to expedite this process. If you are wearing a race belt, spin it around now so your number is on your front.

You will take your bag and run into the changing tent once again. Dump out your run gear and put your bike gear in the bag as you change. Hand this bag to a volunteer or leave it in the changing area and someone will pick it up for you.

How do I get all my transition bags back at the end of the race?

There will be a designated pick-up point where you will collect all of your bags at the finish line.

THE RUN

You finished the swim; you completed the bike. Hopefully you felt great during both legs and hit whatever goals you had set for yourself; process goals, performance goals, or a combination of the two. You took in adequate calories and kept hydrated, you biked within your limitations, and now you are ready to run.

Even through you have done numerous brick workouts in training, your legs will still feel a little funny right out of T2. Take your time and don't blaze out of the transition area. Go out a little slower than normal and let your legs loosen up a bit. Triathletes will often sprint out of T2 from the excitement of finishing the bike and the cheering of the spectators, and this will cost them later. Begin slowly and pick up steam as you go. Remember to try and "negative split" the run, finishing faster than you started. This can be extremely difficult to do, especially in

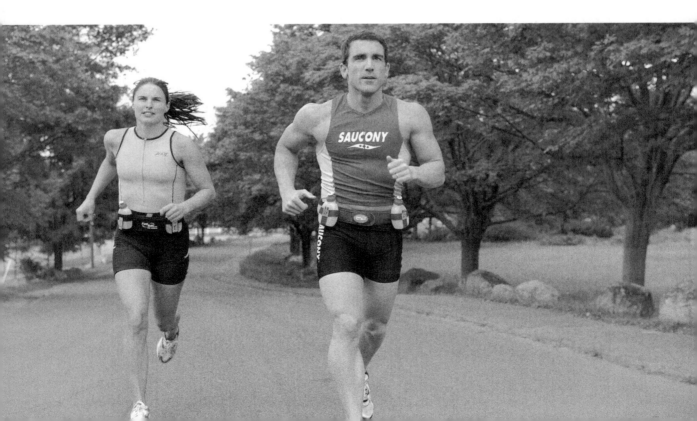

longer triathlons, but if you can master the art of the negative split, you will be way ahead of the game as well as your competition.

Why do people wear hats during the run? I thought wearing a hat would make you hotter in the sun by keeping in your body heat.

Not so. If you will be doing a triathlon in a hot and sunny environment, I highly recommend that you wear a hat. Not a wool cap mind you, or a thick John Deere baseball hat either, but a breathable running cap made specifically for this purpose. It will keep the sun from beating down on your head and will shade your face during the run. You can dump water on it at the aid stations to keep your body temperature even cooler. If you wonder whether wearing a hat is a good thing to do, just watch the Hawaii Ironman on television—it takes place in brutal sun and extreme temperatures and the majority of these elite triathletes are wearing caps during the run.

Once you have warmed up from the transition from the bike, you can start to pick up your run pace if you wish. This is the final leg of your triathlon, after all; you needn't hold back anything for later. Just make sure you don't pick it up too much too soon. How do you know how much to take it up and when? Through experience; trial and error.

Aid Stations

As on the bike course, there will be aid stations periodically along the run course. Both the number of aid stations and what will be provided at each will vary greatly from race to race. Again, it's a good idea to find out what will be available at the aid stations before your race and try to get used to the specific products. These stations are generally a mile or two apart at most triathlons and will most likely have water and a Gatorade-type drink available. Longer races will have more food and drink choices, as outlined earlier. Remember to take in fluids at each station and do not skip any, even if you do not feel thirsty. You should drink at least one full cup at every station, more if it is an extremely hot environment.

Take your time at the aid stations. I recommend walking through them rather than running. Getting in your fluids is too important to potentially miss them or not take in enough while hammering through the aid stations. You can also take this time to pour water over your head to cool down if you are really hot, making sure to keep your feet dry in the process.

Make certain it is water in the cup before you pour it over your head; being covered in sticky Gatorade or Coke for the remainder of your run will not be a pleasant sensation.

I bend over at the waist and pour water on my hat and head as I walk slowly away from the station, making sure the water doesn't hit my shoes. Wet feet are no fun to run in and will blister up fast during longer runs.

If you are wearing a Fuel Belt, be sure to take in your liquid nutrition and salt tablets as you have practiced. I use the Fuel Belt to hold my PowerGels and salt tablets and I get my fluids from the aid stations.

My strategy right now is that I premix two PowerGels with water in each Fuel Belt bottle for my longer triathlons. This way I can take them whenever I want (you want to wash each of your gels down with a few ounces of water to digest them optimally), regardless of where I am on the course. In other words, I take one gel every thirty minutes, and it just might happen that I am not near an aid station when that thirty-minute interval hits. If I don't have any water at that point, it will be harder to take in that gel and the next station might be far off, thus taking me off my schedule. With my gels already mixed, I can keep to my strict plan and take in my fluids in between.

The Run/Walk Method

Made famous by running coach Jeff Galloway, the run/walk strategy involves running for a set period of time, recovering with a walk for a short interval, then repeating this throughout the race. It has become more and more popular during marathons and also for longer-distance triathlons. So, you may run for a mile, walk for thirty seconds, then repeat this for, say, the 13.1 mile run of your Half-Ironman. Some running purists and other people argue that, if you run and walk, you are not a true "runner" or "triathlete." I think this criticism of this race strategy is ludicrous for three main reasons:

1. One of the goals of sports science is to try to find a way to improve performance while exerting less effort. Run/walking achieves this.
2. It is a race. The goal is to get to the finish line as fast as you can within the rules. Run/walking achieves this.
3. It works. This is especially true in longer triathlons, when energy conservation is crucial. You can actually go faster by taking occasional walk breaks because you will end up running faster between these breaks than you would have had you not walked at all.

I have a triathlete friend who recently ran a 2:53 marathon run/walking for 10 seconds every mile. Not too shabby.

Do you have to run/walk during your triathlon? Absolutely not. If you walk through the aid stations as I described earlier, you will actually be doing a form of it without realizing it. Just know that it is an option and can, in fact, improve your times for the longer-distance triathlons. How often and for how long you walk is up to you—just remember that results don't say whether or not you walked, just what your finishing time was.

THE FINISH LINE

As you approach the finish line of your triathlon, check to make sure your race number is flat and can be read easily. They usually take pictures of you as you cross the line and match your pictures with your number. You can usually order the pictures online after the race by going to the race Web site and punching in your name and/or race number on the link for "photos." Smile as you cross the line and raise your arms in the air—you have completed your triathlon!

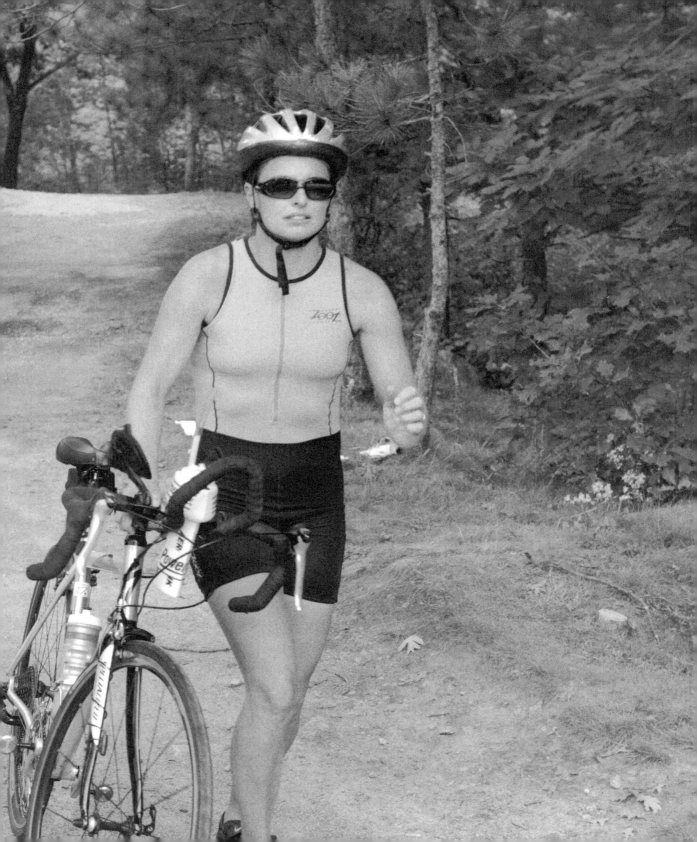

CHAPTER 14
Postrace

The first thing you should do after your race is relax and enjoy your accomplishment. You have dedicated a great deal of time and effort to achieving your goal, and you need to take pride in reaching your goal. If it was your first triathlon, congratulations! Hopefully, you enjoyed the experience of both training and racing and plan on doing more in the future.

Take a few days off from exercise and allow your body to recover from the race. The longer your race, the longer you need to rest. After a few days, you can do a few easy workouts to slowly get back into a routine.

Perhaps you achieved the goals you set for yourself, perhaps not. Reevaluate these goals and see if you set appropriate ones for yourself.

After a few days off, go back and look through your journal and review your training. See if there are any areas where you need improvement. Did you miss a significant number of swim workouts? Did you decide that you didn't want to strength train for triathlon? Or maybe you did more workouts than were assigned and this negatively affected your race performance and enjoyment. Take an objective look at your training notes and begin to plot out how and where you can improve your triathlon performance.

After you have recovered and taken some time to reflect on your accomplishment, I highly recommend setting a new set of goals for yourself. They can be new triathlon race goals—perhaps you want to improve your performance at this distance or maybe you want to try a longer-distance triathlon. Maybe you want to take a little time off from triathlon but would like

★ **THE PMS**

What I have termed the PMS, or Post Marathon Syndrome, applies to triathlon as well; it is the "depression" people tend to fall into after completing their race. They have worked long and hard to achieve their goals and many experience a letdown in the days after their race. This is normal. The secret is to take those few days off right after, to recover and enjoy your accomplishment, then slowly get back into exercising. It need not (and should not) be at the frequency and intensity of your prior training, just enough to keep your body and mind fresh and motivated.

to run some road races instead. Adventure races, organized bike tours, or simply working out a specific number of times per week—all of these are possible future goals that will keep you on the track of fitness. Set new goals for yourself. As I discussed way back at the beginning of this book, if it is a new race you plan on doing, sign up for it, pay the entrance fee, and tell a bunch of your friends that you are doing it.

Triathlon is becoming more and more popular and races are filling up faster and faster as a result. Many of the really popular races fill up in as fast as a few hours, so if you really want to do a particular event, make sure to sign up immediately. Most Ironman races in the United States fill up within a few days, so you have to decide a year ahead of time that you want to compete in one!

Just pick a new fitness goal, big or small, whatever it may be. Continue to take care of your body, test your limits through fitness, and believe in yourself.

At Ironman New Zealand, a Japanese competitor arrived at transition 1 after exiting the water and soon realized that he had forgotten to put his bike shoes in his transition bag. Instead of feeling sorry for himself and quitting, he merely rode off on the 112-mile bike leg with his bare feet on top of the clips, hardly an efficient or pain-free way to pedal, to say the least. Well, he not only finished the bike in an amazingly fast time, but he also hammered through the run as well, and actually ended up qualifying for the Hawaii Ironman at this race, bare feet and all.

Push yourself—you have no idea what you can accomplish or how tough you are until confronted with a challenge.

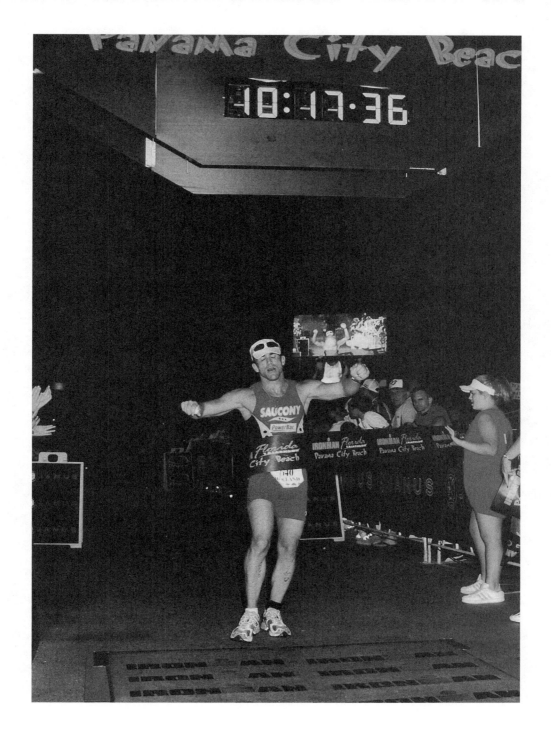

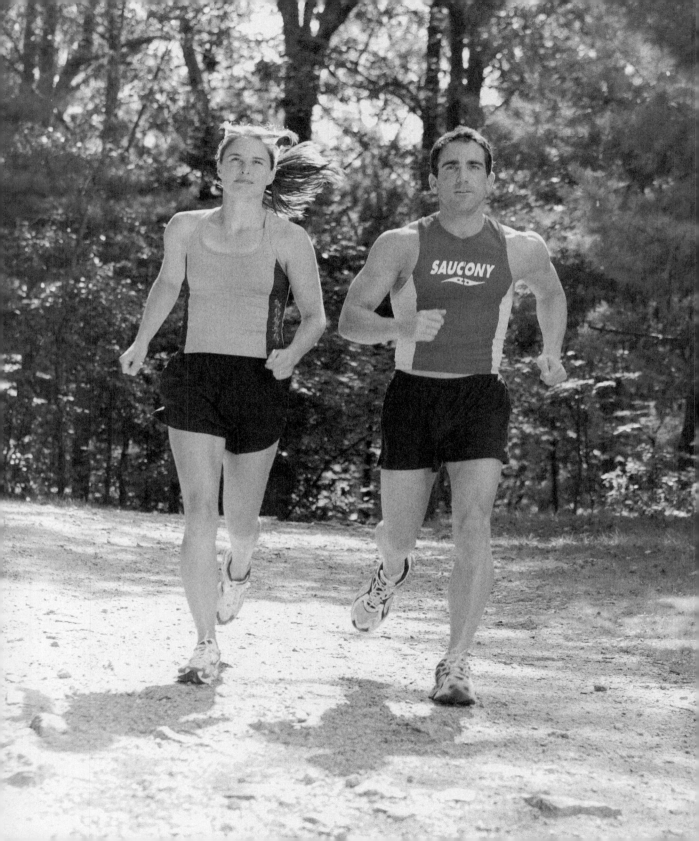

Training Logs

BASE PHASE								
Week		12		11		10		9
Session	1	2	3	4	5	6	7	8
Date								
Dumbbell Chest Presses								
Dumbbell Bent-Over Rows								
Dumbbell Overhead Presses								
Dumbbell Biceps Curls								
Dumbbell Kick Backs								
Stability Ball Squats								
Stationary Lunges								
Stability Ball Hamstring Curls								
Calf Raises								
Dumbbell Toe Raises								
Oblique Twists								
Regular Crunches								
Superman								
Plank								

NOTES:

BUILD PHASE						
Week		8		7		6
Session	9	10	11	12	13	14
Date						
Push-ups						
Dumbbell Bent-Over Rows—Bent Arms						
Dumbbell Alternating Biceps Curls						
Dumbbell Front and Side Raises						
Triceps Bench Dips						
Bench Step Ups						
Front Lunges						
Back Lunges						
Single Leg Calf Raises						
Single Leg Dumbbell Toe Raises						
Double Crunches						
Knee Down Oblique Twists						
Swim						
Raised Leg Plank						
Plank						

NOTES:

PEAK PHASE						
Week		5		4		3
Session	15	16	17	18	19	20
Date						
Stability Ball Push-ups						
Dumbbell Bent-Over Flyes						
Single Leg Stability Ball Squats						
Front and Back Lunges Combo						
Single Leg Stability Ball Hamstring Curls						
Stability Ball Wall Sit						
Stability Ball Reverse Crunches						
Two-Point Bridge						
Plank						

NOTES:

BASE PHASE—WEEK 12							
Day	Monday	Tuesday	Wednesday	Thursday	Friday	Saturday	Sunday
Date							
Swim							
Bike							
Run							
Brick							

NOTES:

BASE PHASE—WEEK 11

Day	Monday	Tuesday	Wednesday	Thursday	Friday	Saturday	Sunday
Date							
Swim							
Bike							
Run							
Brick							

NOTES:

BASE PHASE—WEEK 10							
Day	Monday	Tuesday	Wednesday	Thursday	Friday	Saturday	Sunday
Date							
Swim							
Bike							
Run							
Brick							

NOTES:

BASE PHASE—WEEK 9

Day	Monday	Tuesday	Wednesday	Thursday	Friday	Saturday	Sunday
Date							
Swim							
Bike							
Run							
Brick							

NOTES:

BUILD PHASE—WEEK 8							
Day	Monday	Tuesday	Wednesday	Thursday	Friday	Saturday	Sunday
Date							
Swim							
Bike							
Run							
Brick							

NOTES:

BUILD PHASE—WEEK 7							
Day	Monday	Tuesday	Wednesday	Thursday	Friday	Saturday	Sunday
Date							
Swim							
Bike							
Run							
Brick							

NOTES:

BUILD PHASE—WEEK 6

Day	Monday	Tuesday	Wednesday	Thursday	Friday	Saturday	Sunday
Date							
Swim							
Bike							
Run							
Brick							

NOTES:

PEAK PHASE—WEEK 5

Day	Monday	Tuesday	Wednesday	Thursday	Friday	Saturday	Sunday
Date							
Swim							
Bike							
Run							
Brick							

NOTES:

PEAK PHASE—WEEK 4

Day	Monday	Tuesday	Wednesday	Thursday	Friday	Saturday	Sunday
Date							
Swim							
Bike							
Run							
Brick							

NOTES:

Day	Monday	Tuesday	Wednesday	Thursday	Friday	Saturday	Sunday
Date							
Swim							
Bike							
Run							
Brick							

PEAK PHASE—WEEK 3

NOTES:

TAPER PHASE—WEEK 2							
Day	Monday	Tuesday	Wednesday	Thursday	Friday	Saturday	Sunday
Date							
Swim							
Bike							
Run							
Brick							

NOTES:

TAPER PHASE—WEEK 1

Day	Monday	Tuesday	Wednesday	Thursday	Friday	Saturday	Sunday
Date							
Swim							
Bike							
Run							
Brick							

NOTES:

Helpful Triathlon Web Sites

- www.insideoutsports.com
- www.headsweats.com
- www.ironmanlive.com
- www.runningshoes.com
- www.teamorca.com
- www.insidetri.com
- www.totalimmersion.net
- www.fuelbelt.com
- www.powerbar.com
- www.nytro.com
- www.usatriathlon.org

Tom Holland's Races

March 6, 1999	Ironman New Zealand 13:39
June 27, 1999	Ironman Germany 11:52
May 20, 2000	Ironman California 11:48
July 9, 2000	Hudson Valley Half Ironman Triathlon 5:49
November 4, 2000	Ironman Florida 10:32
January 28, 2001	Ironman Malaysia 13:28
July 8, 2001	Hudson Valley Half Ironman Triathlon 5:13
July 29, 2001	Ironman Lake Placid 11:13
April 7, 2002	Ironman Australia 11:16
June 16, 2002	Escape From Alcatraz Triathlon 3:06
July 27, 2003	Ironman Lake Placid 11:26
November 9, 2003	Ironman Florida 10:17
August 29, 2004	Ironman South Korea 9:36* [swim cancelled due to a typhoon]

ABOUT THE AUTHOR

Tom Holland is the President and Founder of TeamHolland LLC, a fitness consulting company. Through TeamHolland he produces and stars in fitness videos, authors articles and books, delivers lectures, serves as a consultant to the media and works with clients in his specialty fitness camps.

He has appeared on CNN's Headline News and ABC, has lectured for such organizations as the Gatorade Sports Science Institute and the American Medical Athletic Association, and has written for such magazines as *Inside Triathlon*. He has also contributed to such magazines as *Men's Health, Self* and *Fitness*.

He is the author of *The Truth About How to Get in Shape* and is the program designer and star of the Tom Holland Workout fitness video series. He also stars in the Abs Diet Workout.

Tom received his BA from Boston College in Communications and his Master's Degree from Southern Connecticut State University in Exercise Science and Sport Psychology. He has been certified by numerous fitness organizations including the National Strength and Conditioning Association, the American Council on Exercise and the National Academy of Sports Medicine.

An accomplished endurance athlete and a member of PowerBar's Team Elite, Tom has completed 10 Ironman triathlons to date including Malaysia, New Zealand, Australia, Germany and South Korea. He is a veteran of over 500 races from the 5k to ultra marathon and is a Boston Marathon qualifier.

Tom has coached over one thousand clients to achieve their fitness goals. He resides in Connecticut with his wife Philippa and their black labrador retriever Lucy.